The
Blood Pressure
Cure

Also by Robert E. Kowalski

The 8-Week Cholesterol Cure

The 8-Week Cholesterol Cure Cookbook

The Endocrine Control Diet *(with Calvin Ezrin, M.D.)*

Cholesterol & Children

8 Steps to a Healthy Heart

The Type 2 Diabetes Diet Book *(with Calvin Ezrin, M.D.)*

The Revolutionary Cholesterol Breakthrough

The New 8-Week Cholesterol Cure

The Blood Pressure Cure

8 Weeks to Lower Blood Pressure
without Prescription Drugs

Robert E. Kowalski

BICENTENNIAL
1807
WILEY
2007
BICENTENNIAL

John Wiley & Sons, Inc.

Published by John Wiley & Sons, Inc., Hoboken, New Jersey
Published simultaneously in Canada

Wiley Bicentennial Logo: Richard J. Pacifico

Design and composition by Navta Associates, Inc.

The information contained in this book is not intended to serve as a replacement for professional medical advice. Any use of the information in this book is at the reader's discretion. The author and the publisher specifically disclaim any and all liability aris-ing directly or indirectly from the use or application of any information contained in this book. A health care professional should be consulted regarding your specific sit-uation.

For general information about our other products and services, please contact our Customer Care Department within the United States at (800) 762-2974, outside the United States at (317) 572-3993 or fax (317) 572-4002.

Wiley also publishes its books in a variety of electronic formats. Some content that appears in print may not be available in electronic books. For more information about Wiley products, visit our web site at www.wiley.com.

Library of Congress Cataloging-in-Publication Data:

Kowalski, Robert E.
   The blood pressure cure : 8 weeks to lower blood pressure without
prescription drugs / Robert E. Kowalski.
       p. cm.
   Includes bibliographical references and index.
   ISBN: 978-0-470-12416-1 (cloth)
   1. Hypertension—Alternative treatment. 2. Hypertension—Popular works.
I. Title.
   RC685.H8K69 2007
   616.1'3206—dc22

                                                          2006037899

Printed in the United States of America

10 9 8 7 6 5 4 3 2 1

My father passed away on December 5, 1969, from a massive heart attack. Hypertension was one of the major factors contributing to the disease that claimed his life and took him away from us forever. How I wish I could have had more time with him. How I wish he could have met my wife, Dawn, and our children, Ross and Jenny, his grandchildren.

I love him. I miss him. And I hope this book that I dedicate to his memory will help others live and beat cardiovascular disease so they can enjoy the years taken away from him by a disease we're learning more and more about every day.

Contents

Foreword

I had the pleasure of meeting Bob Kowalski in 2004 at the recommendation of Dr. Jack Sternlieb, a common friend and esteemed cardiac surgeon, as well as the founder of the Heart Institute of the Desert in Rancho Mirage, California. Bob's medical history had been well characterized. He suffered a myocardial infarction (heart attack) at the age of thirty-five years, had three-vessel bypass surgery later that same year in 1978, then required a reoperation four-vessel bypass surgery in 1984. Despite this overwhelming burden and genetic predisposition, Bob has done exceptionally well over the last twenty-two years. With great determination and unending intellectual curiosity, Bob has developed a program applicable for all who wish to prevent and treat patients of cardiovascular risk.

Bob Kowalski, an internationally acclaimed medical journalist of more than thirty-eight years, published *The 8-Week Cholesterol Cure* in April 1987 and a complete revision, *The New 8-Week Cholesterol Cure*, in 2002. He was kind enough to provide me with a copy during one of our initial encounters, and I was immediately captivated by his easily understood but comprehensive writing style that appeals to both the lay and the medically educated population alike. Bob's perspective is interesting in that he not only writes as an authority in his field but also as a person who continues to battle cardiovascular disease himself on a daily basis. A testament to his approach is the fact that he has defied statistics. Most medical prefessionals would have quoted him a ten-year survival at the age of thirty-five, having undergone three-vessel bypass surgery in 1978. We are thankful that Bob continues to beat the odds as he relentlessly questions medical dogma, educates, and pioneers new approaches to disease management.

Bob Kowalski encourages medically trained professionals to think outside of the box. We tend to be poorly educated in the nonpharmacological management of disease. As a group, we are often arrogant, dispelling theories and approaches that we are not comfortable with and criticizing them in the name of good medical science. As much money is spent in the United States on nonpharmacological preparations as is spent on traditional pharmaceuticals. In addition, this market continues to grow because it is tremendously appealing to patients who are able to manage diseases naturally without hard-core pharmaceuticals. It is therefore our duty as health-care professionals to be educated in nontraditional neutraceuticals so that we may both understand and better treat our patients. Bob encourages us to do this by presenting clear and concise data.

As a patient, one can only follow Bob's example. He always encourages one to obtain information, educate oneself, fully understand physicians' recommendations, and, most important, work hand in hand and honestly with one's medical professional.

If one were to design an ideal patient, that would be Bob Kowalski. Bob strides through life, savoring the moments, always considering his glass half full. His enthusiasm is infectious, and he is a true delight to interact with. He is a very compliant patient, as long as the recommendations make sense, and is always questioning, always seeking out a better alternative, if possible. With the same gusto and verve, Bob has undertaken another enormous project, that being the comprehensive management of hypertension. This educational tour will take readers through the history of hypertension, its diagnosis, recommendations for management, and contemporary therapies. Even more, Bob will present the holistic approach to hypertension and will have both laypeople and physicians understand novel, natural, and alternative supplements that can, in many instances, negate the necessity for traditional or hard-core pharmaceuticals. Anecdotally, we have all seen patients in our practices who have responded exceptionally well to lifestyle modification, exercise, weight loss, and moderation in alcohol intake. Supplements such as arginine and grape seed extract have been noted to cure hypertension in my practice. These patients are very proud that they have not had to rely on traditional medications to cure their problem. An advocate and a participant in wonderful physician-patient relationships, Bob will be able to guide you, the reader, to a healthier and happier life.

Listen and learn from a man with considerable personal experience who speaks not from anecdote but from personal triumph. Bob's advice is succinct and logical, and his recommendations are very doable. This book will educate and motivate you, as it has done for me. And let's all remember Bob's quote: "You can fight heart disease and win."

Steven Burstein, M.D.
Associate Director, Cardiac Catheterization Laboratories,
Good Samaritan Hospital
Associate Professor of Medicine, UCLA Medical School

Acknowledgments

It would be impossible to list every person who helped me write this book and bring it to publication. So I would like to take this opportunity to thank everyone who assisted with the research process, finding obscure facts and details, and those who inspired me to write the book in the first place.

I have deep gratitude to the hundreds and thousands of medical researchers all over the world who continue to add pieces to the jigsaw puzzle picture of cardiovascular disease. In the months that it took to write and edit this book, not a single week went by that didn't provide an additional insight through a report of a conference I read on the Internet or an article or an editorial in one of the many journals I read regularly. Most of those men and women—the authors of the articles—don't know me and probably have never heard of me, my books, or my personal fight against heart disease. Yet each has touched me very personally and helped me to share his or her information with my readers.

My thanks go specifically to the people who took their valuable time to review chapters, including Steven Burstein, M.D., who graciously wrote the foreword to the book, and Joseph Keenan, M.D., of the University of Minnesota, who has worked with me on a number of my previous efforts as well. Thanks also to Douglas Walsh, D.O., and his son Douglas Walsh Jr., D.O., a family physician and an internist, respectively, in Florida, who spent their time sharing with me their insights in treating men and women with high blood pressure in the real world outside the university medical centers.

Special thanks to my agent, Mitchell Waters of Curtis Brown, Ltd., and my editor, Tom Miller at John Wiley & Sons, for their confidence in me and my book.

Introduction

Suppose you had a crystal ball to see into the future of your health. Let's say that your crystal ball foretold not only the likelihood of major, possibly fatal illnesses but also ways to prevent those problems. Would you take a look? Would you take the steps—especially if they were pretty simple—to avoid those health problems? Most people would. After all, we want the best possible health and the longest, healthiest lives.

I'm one of the very lucky ones. I survived a heart attack and bypass surgery at age thirty-five in 1978 and a second bypass at age forty-one in 1984. In a very real way, I did have that crystal ball, but I just didn't know how to use it back then. My major risk factor was an elevated cholesterol level. I'd known that for years before the heart attack, but in those days the issue of cholesterol and heart disease was controversial. Moreover, there weren't effective ways to get cholesterol down to healthy levels.

Interestingly, as the years have gone by, we've learned that the lower we can get our cholesterol counts, the more we slash the risk of developing heart disease. Medical students in the 1950s learned that "normal" cholesterol levels were a person's age plus 200. It wasn't until the late 1980s that doctors were advising patients to get those levels down to 200. And today we know that when it comes to cholesterol, the lower the better.

This isn't a book about cholesterol, although I'll discuss it in one of the chapters. This book deals with another one of the Big Three risk factors for heart attack and stroke: blood pressure. The third one, by the way, is cigarette smoking. Those three factors are responsible for the vast majority of heart attacks and strokes, although other factors, especially diabetes, come into play as well.

Ironically, the medical community formally recognized the importance of blood pressure, in 1972, long before that of cholesterol, in 1987. But, as with cholesterol, medical researchers have found, only rather recently, that for the most part, the lower your cholesterol level the better. You can expect that blood pressure control and the prevention of high blood pressure, medically termed hypertension, will get increasing attention in the coming years.

The statistics are staggering. One-third of Americans over the age of eighteen—65 million—have at least mild hypertension. For African American women, it's half the population, and for black men it's a major problem as well. At least one-third of people with high blood pressure are not being treated. That means millions and millions of men and women are at risk for a heart attack or a stroke.

Blood pressure numbers previously considered normal in the United States are now given the new designation "prehypertension." Doctors began using that term in 2003 to denote patients whose seemingly okay levels predicted problems down the road. There's our crystal ball again. Doctors can now predict confidently those who will develop full-blown hypertension in the years to come.

Researchers at Boston University reported that over a four-year period, 5.3 percent, 17.6 percent, and 37.3 percent of study participants younger than sixty-five years with optimum, normal, and high-normal blood pressure, respectively, developed hypertension. For those over sixty-five, the likelihood was 16 percent, 25.5 percent, and 49.5 percent. And a mere 5 percent weight gain jacked up the risk of developing hypertension by an additional 20 to 30 percent.

The higher one's blood pressure, the greater that person's risk of having a heart attack or a stroke. That risk gets multiplied by additional factors, including family history, elevated cholesterol levels, diabetes, cigarette smoking, sedentary behavior, overweight and obesity, and other considerations. To make matters worse, high blood pressure appears to increase the risk of developing Alzheimer's disease in later life.

I'm no doubt more aware of cardiovascular disease, a term that lumps together all diseases of the heart and arteries, including heart attack and stroke, than most. That's because, quite literally, I had to fight heart disease to save my own life. My motivation back in 1984 was to survive to raise my two children. The risk of dying from a second bypass surgery, I was told, was five to six times greater than the first operation, owing to a variety of possible complications. The day I heard those statistics from the surgeon scheduled to do that second bypass was my moment of epiphany.

I swore that if I survived I would devote all my capabilities as a trained medical journalist to learning all I could about heart disease in general and cholesterol in particular. That's because I had already quit smoking cigarettes and my blood pressure was considered normal, and because in 1984 more and more medical authorities were coming to the conclusion that cholesterol was a major risk factor. It was in 1987 that the National Institutes of Health, together with the nation's medical organizations, formed the National Cholesterol Education Program to urge all men and women to get their cholesterol levels checked and, if elevated, to get them down.

It was in that same year that I published my book *The 8-Week Cholesterol Cure*, detailing the program I developed to get my own cholesterol levels down from a dangerously high 269 to 184 in just eight weeks without the use of prescription drugs. I'm the guy who put oat bran in the diet in the United States and around the world. It was years later that the U.S. Food and Drug Administration first gave permission for a food manufacturer to make the health claim that oats, along with a low-fat diet, could help prevent heart disease.

Since then I've devoted my life to studying heart disease and the latest developments on how to prevent it. I've applied those principles to my own heart-healthy regimen and have shared them with my readers in my quarterly publication, *The Diet-Heart Newsletter*, and a number of books including a total rewrite of the original *The New 8-Week Cholesterol Cure*.

I've achieved my goal of sticking around long enough to raise my children, who have now graduated from college and are completely on their own. But now I've set the bar higher. I want to be around to play with my grandchildren someday. And I'm happy to report that my doctors, having regularly tested my heart, think I'll be able to do just that. Not to brag, but rather to inspire, I'm in great health, with a completely unlimited life style.

But I continue to tweak my own regimen as I learn new approaches. And that's why the newest, seventh edition of guidelines issued by the Joint National Committee (JNC7) on blood pressure and hypertension in 2003 really caught my attention. For years, I'd thought that my own blood pressure was perfectly fine, and so did the doctors who examined and tested me. The new guidelines, however, labeled me as prehypertensive. At first, I dismissed the stricter limits as being overly cautious. Actually, a lot of physicians reacted the same way. After all, my numbers, typically around 125/80, had been considered normal, and no doctor had ever talked about any need to lower it.

Then I started to read more about the subject. The data were compelling and overwhelming. The lower one's blood pressure, the lower that person's risk of developing cardiovascular disease. And blood pressure measurements previously considered normal actually predicted future elevations and risk.

Coincidentally, the medical community was coming to the same conclusion that the lower one's cholesterol the better. I had accepted that idea years before and did everything I could to keep my levels of the "bad" LDL cholesterol as low as possible and the "good" HDL cholesterol as high as possible. Why shouldn't I view blood pressure with the same aggressive stance?

As with cholesterol control, however, I did not want to take prescription drugs. The JNC-7 guidelines called for lifestyle modifications, including increased exercise and weight control before resorting to those drugs for prehypertensive patients. But I was already very physically active and at a healthy weight. So I started looking for natural, nonprescription approaches, just as I had done nearly two decades earlier for cholesterol control.

While I had studied blood pressure and hypertension rather extensively during my postgraduate physiology training, my first real encounter on a personal level came during a game of golf with my father in 1967. It seemed that he needed to find a tree or a bush on practically every other hole to urinate. It turned out that Dad had been prescribed a drug called a diuretic to control his hypertension, which was extremely severe.

Not much was known about how to prevent heart attacks and strokes back in those days, but high blood pressure was already considered a major culprit. Unfortunately, doctors knew even less about how to control hypertension other than with the first antihypertensive drugs. And, as is still the case today, those drugs had a long list of side effects, not the least of which was the nuisance my father experienced with the need for frequent urination and fatigue. Many, if not most, men had greatly diminished sexual drive, too.

Dad's hypertension, high cholesterol levels, major stress in his life at the time, and the lack of effective countermeasures all conspired against him, and my beloved father died at the age of just fifty-seven in 1969. He and I were very close, and I miss him to this day and always will. Dad would have made a wonderful grandpa, but he never got to meet his grandchildren and bounce them on his knee.

As I said earlier, I'm one of the lucky ones who survived my fight with heart disease. For many, the first symptom is a fatal heart attack. And I intend to stay lucky. But as someone once said, the harder one works at something, the luckier one gets. And so it was that in 2003 I turned my attention to getting my blood pressure lower. I succeeded in doing just that, and now I want to share my findings.

For millions of men and women, following the simple steps I describe in these pages can keep their blood pressure from rising during the coming years. For millions more, this complete program of lifestyle modification and supplementation with completely safe and harmless substances can bring mild to moderate hypertension under control. And for those whose hypertension is so severe that it definitely requires prescription medications, the program can keep dosages as low as possible, thereby limiting side effects and adverse reactions.

As the old song goes, little things mean a lot. Sure, we'll talk about increasing levels of physical activity, controlling weight, quitting smoking, and coping with stress and depression. By themselves, supplements such as grape seed extract, lycopene, CoQ10, and folic acid can provide a small drop in blood pressure. Combining them into a complete program gives a lot of bang for the buck. And I've learned that little tricks, such as taking my daily aspirin tablet at night rather than in the morning, along with a tiny dose of melatonin, helps keep my blood pressure down even lower while I'm asleep.

Then there's the amino acid l-arginine, one of the building blocks of protein available in supplement form, that's one of my secret weapons against blood pressure. L-arginine is the precursor of a gas produced by the lining of the arteries to keep those arteries elastic and flexible. That, in turn, leads to lowered blood pressure, since healthy arteries are more capable of dealing with increased blood flow throughout the day and especially during times of physical or mental stress.

Until recently, however, findings in research laboratories around the world didn't have a practical application, since l-arginine had to be continuously available in the bloodstream. When taken orally, rather than by infusion directly into a vein administered in a hospital, arginine levels quickly increase in the bloodstream but then just as quickly dissipate. The eureka moment came with the development of a sustained-release formulation that keeps arginine at an optimal level in the blood throughout the day and night.

Research at the University of Texas shows that sustained-release arginine allows for greater blood supply to the heart muscle. And subjects in the study experienced lower blood pressure, especially if their numbers were high to begin with.

With all due respect for physicians, and I give them full credit for helping to keep me alive, they're often too quick to reach for the prescription pad without giving safer and more acceptable alternatives a fair chance. Part of it comes from past experience, knowing that simply telling patients to lose weight and consume less salt doesn't do much to bring blood pressure down.

Furthermore, no one should really expect doctors to keep up with every new little discovery, especially when it comes to supplements. Tell the average doctor that a few capsules of grape seed extract or an amino acid will significantly lower blood pressure, and he or she will likely roll his or her eyes.

I remember very well when my book introduced oat bran to the world as a way to lower cholesterol levels. A lot of doctors thought it was hype and hokum. The research was there, but in journals seldom read by practicing physicians.

So don't be surprised if your doctor is more than a little skeptical when you say you want to try the program detailed in this book before you resort to those prescription drugs. That said, hypertension can be so severe that one must bite the bullet and accept the fact that taking prescription drugs may be unavoidable. The end—saving your life—surely justifies the means. I've devoted a chapter to pharmaceutical agents to help you to understand how they work and why certain drugs are better for different individuals. Even then, however, following the program in this book can and will allow you to keep the dosages of those drugs, and their side effects, to a minimum.

Ironically, at least one aspect of blood pressure prevention and control remains controversial and, at the risk of sounding like a heretic, has been greatly exaggerated. That's the role of salt and sodium in the diet. This topic deserves, and gets, a whole chapter in this book. But the essence of the truth is this: not everyone is salt sensitive and will respond positively to salt restriction. And even those who are salt sensitive would have to follow restrictions so severe that results will typically be negligible.

As with most matters, the salt issue isn't black and white but, rather, a shade of gray. Sodium, the offending part of the salt molecule, sodium chloride, is just one of a group of chemical substances in the body called electrolytes. They also include calcium, magnesium, and potassium. The body requires a balance of all the electrolytes. So, rather than merely cutting back on sodium, the trick is to consume more of the others. Research has shown very convincingly that doing so significantly improves blood pressure.

By the time you finish reading this book, you'll have a very good grasp of just what blood pressure and hypertension are. You'll learn that the ideal level is about 115/75. Those numbers reflect blood pressure measured in millimeters of mercury either in your doctor's office or with a home unit. The top number, the systolic, is the pressure of the major and minor arteries at the time the heart beats. The lower number, the diastolic, is a measurement of pressure while the heart is at rest.

As one professor of anatomy told me, we're all as different on the inside as we are on the outside. So I've devoted a chapter to special considerations for men, women, children, and for people of different ages and races. And since diabetic individuals are at particular risk, I've paid extra attention to their needs.

Sure, I'm going to ask you to make some changes in your patterns of eating and physical activity. But I think you'll agree that the suggestions I make won't be radical or unreasonable. Almost no one is willing to completely change his or her life, so this will be more a matter of taking baby steps of change in your life to help get your pressure down to where it belongs and to protect yourself against heart attack and stroke.

As usual, I've experimented with myself and with my family and friends, especially with some of the dietary suggestions. One particular winner is getting into the habit of making fruit smoothies as a quick breakfast. Each smoothie contains four to five servings of fruit, enough to make a dietitian smile for the entire day. Try one and you'll be hooked. Another component of my daily program is a relaxing cup of hot cocoa before bedtime.

It's important to note that none of the supplements that are part of this program have any potential for side effects or adverse reactions. And I've documented each and every suggestion with research studies published in the world's most prestigious medical journals. Both you and your doctor will be very happy with the results you can achieve with this complete program of optimizing your blood pressure.

Did the program work for me? Absolutely! From previous readings in the high 130s/80s my numbers are now as low as 111/68.

In a nutshell, this book's program will show you ways to attain a healthy weight, cope with stress, get the physical activity you need without having to go to the gym, enjoy a delicious diet that actually lowers blood pressure without deprivation, and use newly researched supplements that often can be just as effective as prescription drugs. The concepts are all based on research done at the world's top medical centers and published in the most prestigious journals. And I've had physicians review what I've written to assure absolute accuracy. I've done my part. I've controlled my own blood pressure, and I'm sharing the information I've learned with you. Now it's up to you to do your part.

The foundation of this program is spelled out in the first chapters, in which I explain what blood pressure is, how to most accurately measure it, and lifestyle modifications that include coping with stress, weight control, dietary improvements, physical activity, and so forth. Whether you prefer the natural approach that I advocate or the use of prescription antihypertensive drugs for blood pressure control, that foundation is essential. But you'll find the really exciting and truly revolutionary breakthroughs in natural blood pressure control in chapter 13, "Daily Blood Press Busters," and chapter 14, "The Blood Pressure Cure 5 Secret Weapons." You wouldn't be cheating to jump right to those chapters. That way you can put some of those things to work for yourself immediately.

Got any doubts about whether it's all worth the effort? Just think about everything you love in this life. Taking the pressure off your heart can add years to your life and improve the quality of those years. Yup, it's really worth it.

Recall the image of the crystal ball. You can, indeed, take a look into your future health by learning your blood pressure and cholesterol numbers. And if they are elevated, you can take the steps to get them under control. Your doctor can help, but to a large extent you hold your destiny in your own hands. I took the steps to achieve heart health, and I know that you can, too!

And after reading this book, I know you'll want to stay in touch with the latest developments in heart health in general and blood pressure control in particular. To do so please visit my Web site, www.thehealthyheart.net. It's completely free; no subscription fee is required.

Since 1987, when my first book, *The 8-Week Cholesterol Cure*, was released, I have published a quarterly newsletter, *The Diet-Heart Newsletter*, to keep my readers up to date on the most recent developments in cardiovascular research to prevent heart disease and stroke, information from conferences and seminars in the medical community not typically covered in the mass media, and new heart-healthy foods, supplements, and other products. To receive a complimentary issue and subscription information, simply send a self-addressed, stamped, business-size envelope to: The Diet-Heart Newsletter, P.O. Box 2039, Venice, CA 90294.

PART ONE

The Blood Pressure Problem

1

Hypertension: The Silent Killer

Blood pressure is sort of like the weather. Everyone talks about it, but not enough people do anything about it. It's often called the silent killer because, for the most part, it has no symptoms. Headaches associated with blood pressure are relatively rare. We see hypertension mentioned over and over again as one of the main risk factors for heart attack and stroke. Every time we visit a doctor's office, we get our blood pressure tested. But the sad fact is that while literally millions of men and women have blood pressure levels that put them at risk, most of them don't get their numbers under control.

I think there are two reasons for this. First, most of us don't understand blood pressure well enough to appreciate its importance. Second, many people aren't willing to take drugs that carry a heavy load of side effects or they don't want to make what they think will be major lifestyle sacrifices to eliminate a risk factor that doesn't appear to really bother them. In this book, you'll learn everything you need to know about blood pressure and you'll be delighted to find out that most people who have mild to moderate blood pressure elevations don't have to take prescription drugs or make major changes in their lives.

You already know more about blood pressure than you realize. That's because you're very familiar with the plumbing in your own house. One of life's great pleasures is taking a shower with water gushing powerfully over your body. That comes from having sufficient water pressure in your bathroom pipes. You also need good water pressure to wash the dishes, water the lawn, and wash the car. Conversely, we all know the frustration of having low water pressure. We might even have to call the plumber if the pressure falls too low. He'll use a little device to measure the pressure at different points in the house and the yard and make suggestions as to how you can improve the situation. Maybe mineral deposits have clogged the plumbing. Once the problem or problems are fixed, you can have water pressure on demand.

That's pretty easy to understand, right? We can all relate to that scenario. Well, it's really not so different from the way blood pressure works. When we're young, our arteries—our internal pipes—are flexible and elastic and allow blood flow to be controlled without any problem. But as we age, and owing to other causes, our arteries stiffen and are unable to dilate and constrict adequately to provide our bodies with enough blood and oxygen. This explains 90 percent of cases of hypertension, medically referred to as primary hypertension. In African Americans, an increase in blood output when the heart's ventricle pumps also plays an important role, as does their greater sensitivity to salt and sodium. Going back to the water pipe analogy, the development of hypertension is a gradual process that we scarcely notice. Tragically, the first "symptom" might be a heart attack or a stroke. I've written this book to help to prevent such a tragic occurrence in your life.

So, enough about those water pipes. What about blood pressure? We'll start with the heart, which is essentially a marvelously designed chunk of muscle and chambers that pumps blood through an extensive network of arteries to every tissue in the body. Blood then returns to the heart through a parallel system of veins, where it collects in two chambers called the atria. Valves permit that blood to enter the other two chambers, the ventricles. Blood leaving the heart has been oxygenated by the lungs and brings that oxygen to our muscles and other tissues. When blood returns, it is reoxygenated and gathers in the atria. Then the heart's left ventricle forcefully pumps oxygenated blood out through the aorta and on to the rest of the body's arteries.

Blood pressure is the force of our blood pushing against the walls of our arteries. As our hearts beat, typically 60 to 70 times a minute when we're sitting or lying down, blood is forced into and through the arteries. Blood pressure is highest when the heart beats, pumping that blood. That's the systolic pressure. Between beats, when the heart is at rest, blood pressure falls. That's the diastolic pressure. Blood pressure is expressed as the systolic pressure over the diastolic pressure, as in 120 over 80, written as 120/80. In the next chapter we'll go into detail about how blood pressure is tested and how those numbers are determined.

There are three known methods by which the body controls blood pressure. First are the pressure receptors in various organs that can detect changes in blood pressure and then adjust the pressure by altering both the force and the speed of the heart's contractions, as well as the total resistance to pressure. Second, the kidneys are responsible for the long-term adjustment of blood pressure through a system involving various chemical substances in the so-called renin-angiotensin system. Third, in response to high levels of either potassium or angiotensin, the steroid aldosterone is released from the adrenal glands, one of which is located on top of each kidney. This hormone then increases the excretion of potassium by the kidneys, while also increasing sodium retention in the body. For most of my readers, this information is far more than they need, but I provide it here for people with some medical background.

What happens, though, when the arteries, an essential part of our cardiovascular systems, fail to perform optimally? Let's say that a woman finds herself under heavy emotional stress. A man goes out in the winter to shovel snow that fell during the night. A fairly young guy decides to play in a pick-up game of basketball after too many years of a sedentary lifestyle. In all three cases, the heart beats faster to pump out more blood than usual, but the arteries aren't up to the task. They are unable to convey the necessary blood to the heart and the brain because they can't dilate enough to accommodate the larger-than-usual blood volume. Pressure increases on the walls of the arteries, but the arteries just can't open up enough. In addition, plaque may rupture, spilling its contents into the bloodstream, which precipitates the formation of a large blood clot. The result is a heart attack or a stroke. The aftermath of a stroke can be devastating for people who survive. While heart attacks and strokes most typically involve a number of factors, extreme hypertension, medically termed *malignant*, can alone be responsible.

Okay, enough of the potentially tragic devastation of life. The good news is that most such heart attacks and strokes can be prevented by controlling, by "curing," the risk factors that cause them. The more we learn, the better the news gets. Based on data from the National Health and Nutrition Examination Survey in the United States, an ongoing decades-long evaluation, as many as three out of four cardiovascular events could be prevented by optimal control of blood pressure and cholesterol. That conclusion came from studying the data from 1,921 people ages thirty to seventy-four. Interestingly, this dramatic saving of lives could be accomplished from bringing blood pressure down to levels that most doctors still believe to be too high, no more than 140/90. This book will show you how to get those numbers down much lower, improving your odds even more.

As early as 1957, the Metropolitan Life Insurance Company published a chart showing that as blood pressure levels rose, life expectancy fell. Conversely, the lower the levels, the longer the life. And who doesn't want a long, healthy life?

For decades hypertension, or high blood pressure, has been recognized as one of the Big Three risk factors for cardiovascular disease, along with elevated cholesterol levels and cigarette smoking. With what we know today, though, diabetes should be added to the list of major risk factors—one of the Big Four. Of course, genes and family medical history play a huge role, but those genetic traits simply predispose you to problems down the road. Eliminate the risk factors that convert the potential to the real, and the question of family history becomes virtually moot. When I began preaching that mantra twenty years ago, many doctors said I was exaggerating, oversimplifying. Back in 1978, actuarial tables that predicted life span indicated death within ten years for a man of thirty-five who had a family history of cardiovascular disease, had a long list of risk factors, and had suffered a heart attack and undergone bypass surgery. This means that I should have been dead by age forty-three, sooner rather than later. But I guess I fooled them! Today the vast majority of doctors and medical authorities agree that cardiovascular diseases, and deaths from heart attacks and strokes, are largely preventable. You simply have to make the decision, as I did, to eliminate the risk factors. As virtually any doctor will tell you, the risk posed by hypertension can be completely eliminated.

Here's a happy thought, something to inspire your commitment to good health in general and to blood pressure control in particular. Several—not just one or two—trials have demonstrated without doubt that reductions of systolic blood pressure by as little as one to three points will decrease your relative risk of stroke by as much as 20 to 30 percent. That's one heck of a return on your investment!

The following numbers speak for themselves, and I present them without commentary or fearmongering. Statistics from the American Heart Association in 2006 show that 65 million men and women in the United States have high blood pressure, defined as systolic pressure of 140 or greater and/or diastolic pressure of 90 or more. In the white population, 20.5 percent have hypertension, while that percentage jumps to 31.6 for African Americans. Nineteen percent of Hispanics and 16.1 percent of Asians have hypertension.

These rates of high blood pressure contribute significantly to the annual occurrences of 7.2 million heart attacks and 5.5 million strokes—pretty scary numbers. But there's a lot we can do to make sure we're not counted in those statistics.

Hypertension Risk Factors and What We Can Do about Them

Family history certainly plays a large role in determining whether you will develop hypertension, but I prefer to think of it merely as a warning. If the gate goes down and the lights go on at a railway crossing, you've got a pretty good idea that a train is on its way. A wise person would never put himself or herself in harm's way by trying to race a car across the tracks. We don't tempt fate by indulging in reckless behavior. Just because your grandfather had hypertension and died from a stroke doesn't mean that you can't take steps to avoid repeating that history.

Race definitely comes into play. High blood pressure is far more common in blacks than in any other racial group, and it hits at an earlier age. But we know that African Americans are far more sodium sensitive than whites are and at the same time they have diets that are high in sodium, doubling the problem. The solution seems pretty obvious. Similarly, obesity and diabetes are more prevalent among blacks. Rather than wringing his or her hands in despair, the wise black individual will take appropriate action.

High blood pressure is more common in young and middle-aged men than in women of similar ages. In those age sixty and older, however, it is more common in women. Blood pressure testing, a simple and painless way to know if you're at risk, is available to everyone, regardless of sex.

You can certainly take control of the other risk factors involved in the gradual progression of elevated blood pressure and subsequent hypertension. Obesity plays a big part. The greater your body mass, the more blood is needed to supply oxygen and nutrients to your muscles and other tissues. Obesity increases the number and length of blood vessels, thereby increasing the resistance of blood that has to travel longer distances through those vessels. Increased resistance results in higher blood pressure. Fat cells themselves manufacture substances that adversely affect both the heart and the blood vessels.

Sedentary behavior boosts your risk by deconditioning the heart muscle just as much as it does other muscles in the body. Couch potatoes tend to have higher heart rates because their heart muscles aren't as efficient and have to work harder to pump blood. Moreover, physical activity is a vasodilator; that is to say, exercise of any sort dilates blood vessels. Combining inactivity with being overweight multiplies the problem.

Sodium and salt intake remain controversial as risk factors for hypertension. While it's true that some individuals are particularly sensitive to sodium, whether from the salt shaker or from sodium-based ingredients in processed and fast foods, not everyone responds to sodium equally. As we'll see, sodium is but one of many minerals, or electrolytes, that affect blood pressure. Increasing your intake of the others may be as important as, or more important than, decreasing your intake of sodium, other than for people who are proven to be sodium sensitive.

Alcohol definitely affects blood pressure, but this is a gray zone. Excessive alcohol consumption can raise blood pressure, whereas moderate drinking may actually help to keep it under control.

Stress is another highly controversial subject in the medical research community, although doctors in clinical practice regularly see the effects of stress in their patients. Stress boosts the production of harmful substances, increases the heart rate and blood requirements, and can over time raise blood pressure and precipitate a heart attack or a stroke. Again, there are many effective, proven methods to help you cope with stress.

Symptoms of High Blood Pressure

For the most part, hypertension is indeed a silent killer with no symptoms to tip you off that something might be wrong. An exception would be someone who experiences a dull headache, typically in the back of the head and usually in the morning. Bear in mind that such headaches are the rare exception rather than the rule.

Ordinary headaches, dizziness, and nosebleeds are not symptoms, at least in the early stages of blood pressure elevation. Those symptoms can occur, however, with severe hypertension. That said, even people with very high blood pressure normally don't have any symptoms.

Because blood pressure is influenced by a waterfall sequence of chemical substances in the kidneys, and because severely high blood pressure can damage the kidneys, certain symptoms may occur in advanced disease states that are not directly caused by blood pressure but rather are due to the damaged kidneys. These include excessive perspiration, muscle cramps, weakness, frequent urination, and a rapid or irregular heartbeat.

Blood Pressure Classification

There has been considerable worldwide discussion, if not controversy, over the classification of increasing levels of blood pressure. That was precipitated in 2003 by the Joint National Committee (JNC) on Blood Pressure and Hypertension, a branch of the National Institutes of Health in the United States. Its seventh set of guidelines for classification and treatment (JNC7) created what future medical historians might ultimately view as a revolutionary landmark in addressing the vital importance of blood pressure control at virtually all levels. Critics, however, both within and outside of the United States, consider JNC7 to be inflammatory and unnecessary. I'll discuss the nuances and I'll let you judge for yourself, viewed from your vantage point as patient, physician, or both.

Following is the categorization of blood pressure and hypertension as defined by the JNC7 report and guidelines.

Category	Systolic	Diastolic
Optimal	115 or less	75 or less
Normal	Less than 120	Less than 80
Prehypertension	120 to 139	80 to 89
Stage 1 hypertension	140 to 159	90 to 99
Stage 2 hypertension	More than 160	More than 100

If either the systolic (upper) or the diastolic (lower) number is in one of the three categories above normal, overall the patient is considered to be in that category.

"Why the big deal? What's the difference?" you might well ask. As I'll detail shortly, the risk of cardiovascular disease, heart attack, stroke, and death rises linearly with blood pressure. Anything more than 120/80 begins to increase the risk, especially when other risk factors are concurrently present, such as elevated cholesterol, cigarette smoking, and especially diabetes. The data are compelling. As you read through them, you'll no doubt prefer to be at the low end of the risk spectrum. Doctors have sometimes been accused of not being aggressive enough in confronting and battling disease, especially degenerative disease that takes a long time to develop. Not anymore!

The biggest point of dissension was the introduction of the term *prehypertension*. With some justification, critics feared that labeling patients as having "prehypertension" rather than "high normal" blood pressure would make them fearful. Some people were concerned that such a label on a medical record might influence medical insurance rates. Others worried that antihypertensive drugs might be prescribed excessively, even though the JNC7 guidelines call for lifestyle modifications before prescribing drugs.

When I first read the JNC7 guidelines, I sided with the critics. But the more I thought about it, the more I agreed that stricter guidelines were better. Interestingly, I had adamantly criticized U.S. cholesterol guidelines for years, complaining to my readers that it was ridiculous to have two sets of guidelines, one for people without cardiovascular disease and another for those who had had a confirmed diagnosis or who had suffered a cardiovascular event of one sort or another. Wouldn't it be better to recommend that everyone get his or her low-density lipoprotein (LDL) as low as possible and high-density lipoprotein (HDL) as high as possible to *prevent* development of the disease or suffering an event rather than waiting for that to happen?

So it is with blood pressure. The lower we can get our numbers, the better off we are now and will be in the future. It really doesn't matter whose chart you're looking at, in Australia, the United States, or elsewhere in the world. All cardiologists and medical authorities agree that your goal should be 120/80 or, even better, down as low as 115/75 or lower.

For many years, doctors believed that diastolic blood pressure, the lower number, was the more important evaluation. Today we know that the opposite is true. Elevations of systolic blood pressure, the top number, are far more predictive of cardiovascular disease that can lead to a heart attack or a stroke. Japanese research published in the journal *Hypertension* in November 2006 documented that elevations in systolic blood pressure are the most predictive of a stroke. According to current hypertension management guidelines, a 5-point reduction in systolic blood pressure can reduce mortality substantially and cut the risk of having a stroke by 14 percent and of getting heart disease by 9 percent. Perversely, systolic blood pressure is far more difficult to lower effectively than diastolic blood pressure. The program components of *The Blood Pressure Cure* have been clinically documented to significantly reduce systolic pressure and therefore your risk of having a heart attack or a stroke.

Pulse pressure is another important consideration for you and your physician. Pulse pressure is essentially the difference between the systolic and diastolic pressure readings. Dr. John Cockcroft, an international authority on blood pressure and hypertension at the University of Wales College of Medicine in the United Kingdom, provided a dramatic example of this in an interview featured on *Medscape Cardiology*, an Internet service for cardiologists and others specializing in heart health. He explained that if you look at the risk of a cardiovascular event such as a heart attack or a stroke in people with a rise of about 20 mm Hg in systolic blood pressure, the risk is not as great as that from a 20 mm Hg rise in pulse pressure. Dr. Cockcroft said that pulse pressure is often a far better predictor of risk than either systolic or diastolic blood pressure alone.

But that doesn't mean you or I should turn into neurotics about our blood pressure levels, which the critics fear might happen. Life is to be lived and enjoyed. Happily, a lot of the things we can do to benefit our blood pressure will make our lives even longer and more enjoyable!

The Rationale for Lower Blood Pressure

The data indicating that the higher the blood pressure, even within limits previously considered completely normal or high-normal, the greater the risk of cardiovascular disease, stroke, heart attack, and death have been building up for several years. These data have reached critical mass, and now virtually all physicians and medical authorities agree that the lower a person can bring his or her blood pressure into an optimal zone of about 115/75 or even less, the better. It now appears that, especially for people over fifty, the systolic (top) number is most important. Even if the diastolic (bottom) number is quite normal, attention should be paid to getting the systolic pressure down. There is a condition termed *isolated systolic hypertension*, in which diastolic pressure is relatively normal but systolic pressure is elevated. Doctors treat that condition aggressively.

In a study at the University of North Carolina involving about nine thousand men and women over a period of 11.6 years, the rate of cardiovascular disease increased significantly as blood pressure levels increased. Compared with patients who had optimal blood pressure levels, those with high-normal measurements had two and a half times the risk of developing cardiovascular disease. That statistic took into consideration other factors involved in the disease. Most of the risk was in the form of a stroke. The risk was greatest for African Americans, diabetics, overweight and obese individuals, and people with high levels of LDL cholesterol.

Researchers concluded that the "prehypertension population is large," and that efforts to lower blood pressure to optimal levels "have the potential to make a significant impact."

Subsequent investigations have proved that to be absolutely true. In a recently published study, nearly nine thousand middle-aged adults with blood pressure levels previously considered to be normal or high normal were broken into three groups and tracked for an average of twelve years. Blood pressure levels in the three groups were: (1) lower than 120/80, (2) 120–129/80–84, and (3) 130–139/85–89. Compared with the group that had the lowest blood pressure, the second and third groups had 70 percent and 144 percent greater risk, respectively, for coronary heart disease.

Moreover, high-normal blood pressure often quickly progresses to frank hypertension within a period of four years or less. The older one is, the greater that risk. In a study at Boston University, nearly half of all adults sixty-five or older who had high-normal blood pressure went on to develop hypertension during that time. And the likelihood of developing hypertension was increased an additional 20 to 30 percent for those who gained an additional 5 percent of body weight. Results were similar in both men and women. Researchers concluded that high-normal blood pressure is more similar to hypertension than it is to normal blood pressure. In other words, there is a continuum.

Here's another sobering statistic from the U.S. JNC7 report. The higher the blood pressure, the greater the risk. For individuals forty to seventy years of age, each increment of 20 mm Hg in systolic blood pressure or 10 mm Hg in diastolic blood pressure *doubles* the risk of cardiovascular disease across the entire blood pressure range from 115/75 to 185/115 mm Hg. Let's put that into some specifics. Let's say your systolic blood pressure increases from 115 to 135 over a period of time. Your risk has been doubled. Over the coming years, if the systolic pressure goes up by another 20 mm Hg to 155, your risk is doubled again. It's a very slippery slope! But the good news is that the opposite also applies. There is a continuous benefit as blood pressure goes down closer and gets closer to that optimal level of 115/75. That should be everyone's target, the holy grail of heart health.

We already know the benefits that can be derived from lowering levels of what is now called prehypertension to more optimal counts. Results of the study known as TROPHY (TRial Of Preventing Hypertension) were presented at the March 2006 meeting of the American College of Cardiology (ACC). The mean age of patients with prehypertension was 48.5 years; half were treated and the other half were not. At the end of the two-year trial, treatment was shown to reduce the risk of progression to hypertension by 66 percent.

In the TROPHY study, treated patients received the antihypertensive drug candesartan. But success can be achieved by lifestyle changes alone, as proved by a project funded by the National Heart, Lung, and Blood Institute of Health. Lifestyle changes that protected the subjects in that study from progressing from prehypertension to hypertension included weight loss, physical activity, moderation of alcohol consumption, and a diet rich in fruits, vegetables, and whole-grain cereals. In fact, an editorial accompanying the report published in the *New England Journal of Medicine* questioned the use of potent pharmacological agents and suggested aggressive lifestyle modification as the superior approach. And that doesn't even take into consideration the use of newly developed, natural supplements clinically documented to lower blood pressure. I discuss those secret weapons later in this book.

International readers might well comment, "Okay, that's the American point of view. But it doesn't necessarily apply to us in other countries." Sorry, but that's just not true. It would get boring, but I could cite study after study from countries around the world, including the United Kingdom, Sweden, Italy, Germany, Finland, and Australia, coming to the same inevitable conclusion: if you want to protect yourself from cardiovascular disease, stroke, heart attack, heart failure, and kidney disease, get your blood pressure down to that optimal 115/75 level or at least as close as possible. That's especially true for people with other risk factors, including elevated cholesterol levels, a family history of cardiovascular disease and premature death, cigarette smoking, diabetes, overweight, a sedentary lifestyle, and unmanaged stress and emotional distress.

2

Testing Your Pressure

To get the best performance and the longest life out of the tires on your car, you want to maintain the rcommended air pressure. To find out whether your tires are at the optimal pressure, you do a simple test or you have the service station do so. The same applies to the pressure on your heart and in your arteries. The first step is to have a simple, painless test done in your doctor's office.

Most men and women have had their blood pressure measured at one time or another. But, bearing in mind that without knowing it, many individuals have either pressure above optimal levels or frank hypertension, if you haven't had a test lately, call your doctor's office and schedule an appointment. While you're there, it would be a good idea to have your cholesterol levels checked as well. Elevated cholesterol counts are not only a major risk factor for heart attack and stroke, in and of themselves, but they also predispose a person to developing hypertension.

To test blood pressure, the doctor or another health professional inflates a cuff placed around the arm above the elbow. He or she then listens for specific sounds through a stethoscope placed at the crook of the elbow as the cuff is gradually deflated. The first of those sounds signals the time the heart beats and the fifth and final sound notes the heart at rest between beats. The pressure at the time of those two sounds is noted in a column of mercury similar to that in a thermometer, on a device called a sphygmomanometer, which is frequently mounted on the wall. The first, beating pressure is termed systolic (the upper number as in 120/80) and the second is diastolic. Both are measured in millimeters of mercury (mm Hg).

Some medical offices now use a digital apparatus to test blood pressure, reducing the environmental impact of mercury. But the mercury sphygmomanometer is still considered the gold standard and is used to calibrate the accuracy of other devices.

Many things affect blood pressure, so it's best to have at least two and preferably three measurements done while you're in the doctor's office. To make a diagnosis of hypertension, rather than merely of somewhat elevated levels, the doctor should test your blood pressure during three separate office visits.

Here are a few things you can do to make sure your test is as accurate as possible. Get a good night's sleep the night before your visit. Wear a shirt or a blouse that can be easily rolled up on the arm so the cuff can be placed on bare skin. Sit with both feet on the floor. Ideally, relax for a few minutes before the test by taking a few deep breaths and thinking happy thoughts. If you're in the doctor's office for some other reason, ask to have your pressure measured at the end, rather than the start, of your appointment.

Smoking and drinking caffeinated beverages can raise blood pressure for two or more hours. Conversely, older people's pressure might be lower immediately after eating. It may be higher in the morning than in the afternoon or the evening. Talking tends to make pressure go up, so it's best to remain silent during the test.

It's natural to have a certain amount of anxiety before any test, and this might make the pressure higher. That's why it's best to have more than one measurement taken during your visit. Wait a few minutes after the first measurement, then have the test repeated, ideally a couple of times.

White Coat, Labile, and Masked Hypertension

A lot of people, including myself, naturally have a bit of anxiety when visiting the doctor's office. As a result, blood pressure may well be higher in that setting than when at home. Such elevations are called "white coat hypertension." Often pressure will go down during the course of the visit, but not always. That's one reason home monitoring is getting more popular with both patients and doctors. We'll get into testing yourself in more detail later.

Researchers in Japan investigated white coat hypertension (WCH) in 128 subjects. At home, their blood pressure levels on average were 135/85. In the doctor's office they rose to 140/90. Many men and women experience even greater differences.

In a study at the University of Virginia, systolic blood pressure (top number) was an average of 14 points higher in patients who were tested shortly after arriving in the exam room while seated on the examining table than in those who sat for five minutes in a chair. Doctors believe that foot and back support help one to relax and that more accurate readings result.

Until recently, medical authorities considered WCH to be benign. The Japanese investigators wondered whether WCH might signal the future development of actual hypertension. Over a period of eight years, they compared patients with WCH with those whose blood pressure was normal in the doctor's office. Nearly twice as many WCH patients went on to develop hypertension as did people with normal blood pressure. Risk of future hypertension was greater for men and for older and/or overweight individuals.

There are no known biochemical, physiological, or personality predictors of WCH. That means neither you nor your doctor can tell whether you're one of at least 10 percent of the population whose blood pressure will be higher in the office than at home.

Interestingly, even people who are being treated for hypertension and whose blood pressure is controlled by drugs can experience WCH. That was proved to be the case by medical investigators in Greece, who compared the responses of hypertensive patients with those of subjects who had normal blood pressure. They suggested monitoring outside the clinical setting.

Blood pressure similarly rises with anxiety and stress during everyday life. That's a natural and usually harmless phenomenon. You're driving along the road, let's say, and a child runs out into the street and you slam on the brakes. Your blood pressure goes up as a normal response, but it's also normal for your blood pressure to return to stress-free levels after a few minutes.

Some individuals, however, have a condition called "labile hypertension," in which blood pressure stays up longer than it should. Those men and women are likely to experience increases in blood pressure more frequently than others, responding more dramatically to the stress and anxiety that everyone has to one degree or another.

As with WCH, labile hypertension (LH) wasn't considered dangerous in the past, but it now sends a signal to doctors that the person is more likely than others are to develop full-blown hypertension. While it's true that there are no symptoms of hypertension or high blood pressure, we all know when we're angry or frightened or would like to shoot someone. These emotional states elevate blood pressure. The question is, how long does that pressure stay up? The two ways of answering that question are home monitoring and ambulatory monitoring, wearing a device that continuously records blood pressure through a twenty-four-hour period. Again, more about those later.

Last, we have individuals whose blood pressure appears normal when they're in the doctor's office but goes up outside the clinical setting. Such people suffer from "masked hypertension." They are more likely to be male, be young, and have higher than normal heart rates, according to Israeli researchers. They suggest that masked hypertension (MH) may be caused, at least in some cases, by a high level of physical activity during the day. In the Israeli study, 11 percent of subjects exhibited MH.

As with WCH and LH, MH is best revealed by monitoring blood pressure either with occasional home monitoring or by wearing an ambulatory device provided by a physician who, for whatever reason, suspects MH. MH is also known in the medical community as "reverse white coat hypertension" and "white coat normotension." This is particularly insidious, since such patients tend to be at even greater risk than are people with more commonly detected hypertension.

Factors Affecting Blood Pressure Readings

Levels of blood pressure vary significantly through the day and night. The lowest pressures occur during sleep. Conversely, virtually everyone has, to one degree or another, what is termed *morning surge* in blood pressure.

Doctors have noted this tendency for many years, but the definitive study was done in 2003. Investigators from the United States and Japan collaborated in the work that determined that significant morning surges in blood pressure present a major risk of stroke for older patients with hypertension. Previous work established a similar risk for older people arising from an afternoon siesta. It's scary to think that taking a nap can actually be hazardous to one's health!

Morning surge is now medically defined as the difference in systolic blood pressure during the first two hours after awakening and arising minus the lowest level of systolic blood pressure recorded during the day or, ideally, during sleep. The greater the difference, the higher the risk of stroke. In the 2003 study, people at the highest risk had a whopping difference averaging 55 mm Hg.

Please note that the risk of stroke was increased for older patients with established hypertension, *not* for those with normal or minimally elevated blood pressure. Older hypertensive individuals, however, should be aware of this risk and should determine with either home or ambulatory monitoring whether they experience morning surge.

Even the weather affects blood pressure. Daytime blood pressure tends to be lower during the hot days of summer than during cold weather. That's true regardless of age, but older men and women with hypertension have higher blood pressure at night when the weather is hot. Such individuals are typically treated with antihypertensive drugs to control their blood pressure, and they and their doctors should be aware that just because blood pressure might be measured as being lower in the summer days, their medication dosages should not be reduced.

Home and Ambulatory Blood Pressure Monitoring

Technology has taken great strides forward during the last decade or longer. Most people today have access to a computer and many of us use one every day. Giant TV screens dominate family rooms, turning them into home theaters with DVD players. Cell or mobile telephones are everywhere, linking friends, family, and businessmen and professionals wherever they go.

Ten years ago, doctors scoffed at the idea of measuring and monitoring blood pressure at home rather than in the medical office. Today many physicians, at least those in the know, recognize that modern home blood pressure monitors are as good as, or perhaps even better than, clinical testing. That trend is worldwide.

Late in 2004, the American Heart Association advocated home monitoring in its revised guidelines for blood pressure measurements, published in the February 2005 issue of the journal *Hypertension*. The lead author of that report, Dr. Thomas Pickering of Columbia University in New York, said, "We've found that blood pressure measurements taken by doctors in their offices may actually be unreliable in many patients. For that reason, there is wider acceptance of blood pressure readings taken by patients in their homes, and of ambulatory blood pressure monitoring."

Greek medical researchers found that home monitoring is actually superior to both clinical testing and ambulatory monitoring. They systematically tested and compared the three methods over a three-month period of time in 133 patients. The team determined that home monitoring produced the most accurate measurements. They wrote that such monitoring would lead to better success with prescription drugs to lower blood pressure, but this also applies, of course, to natural, nonprescription techniques of maintaining normal blood pressure and lowering elevated levels.

Not only were early home monitors inaccurate, but they were also expensive. Today they are both accurate and inexpensive. They're a great investment in cardiovascular health for you and the entire family. Even children? Authorities advocate blood pressure testing for people who are at least eighteen. And if there's a family history of heart disease, hypertension, and stroke, it's a good idea to start as young as thirteen. By the way, that also applies to testing for cholesterol levels. Because of my own battle with heart disease and my family history, I made a heart-healthy lifestyle a family affair well before my children entered their teens.

You'll find many brands of blood pressure monitors in the marketplace. Two excellent choices are Omron and LifeSource, both certified accurate by the British Hypertensive Society, internationally recognized for evaluating blood pressure monitoring devices. Omron is more widely distributed and is very respected. LifeSource has some extra features, including an indicator of cardiac arrhythmias, or heartbeat disturbances, on certain models. You can find Omron in pharmacies, discount stores, and online. Check out LifeSource as well at www.lifesourceonline.com. You'll be happy with either product.

I personally believe that a home blood pressure monitoring device should be as common in households as bathroom scales are to keep track of weight. When clothing feels tight, one can assume that he or she has gained weight. But since blood pressure elevations usually have no symptoms, only regular monitoring can let us know that our blood pressure is in the healthy range.

Even though the home monitoring devices are extremely easy to use, technique is important to assure accurate blood pressure measurements. It's best to sit at a table or a desk, wrap the cuff around the arm as directed in the instructions, and relax for a couple of minutes before inflating the cuff. Keep both feet on the floor and try to remain still, since movement can decrease accuracy. Your arm and cuff should be at the same height as your heart. Hit the start button and note your blood pressure. Many machines also measure heart rate. Wait a couple more minutes and repeat the procedure. You'll probably find that the first measurement is higher.

To establish what doctors call a baseline, keep a chart of your blood pressure measurements at various times of the day. Jot down a few notes. Was it a hot day? Were you under a lot of stress? Did you have a lot of coffee to drink that day? An alcoholic beverage? Do that for a week. Then periodically retest your blood pressure. If it was elevated and you begin to follow the suggestions in this book, you'll be pleased to see improvements in the coming weeks and months!

You'll want to share your data with your doctor. It's a good idea to have your machine calibrated in his or her office, comparing the measurements you get on your home device with the mercury-based sphygmomanometer in the clinical setting.

What about the ambulatory blood pressure monitoring (ABPM) I've referred to? This employs an apparatus provided by the physician and provides a twenty-four-hour record of blood pressure levels, with readings taken at fifteen- to thirty-minute intervals throughout the day and night. ABPM is used for patients with white coat hypertension, to determine whether morning surges are occurring, to measure blood pressure during sleep, and to learn how well antihypertensive drugs are working. Typically, ABPM is prescribed for patients with severe hypertension, especially for older people. ABPM is becoming more popular among hypertension experts as being the most definitive method to truly determine a patient's risk. ABPM allows a doctor to determine the average blood pressure throughout the day, a more informative measurement than a few tests at the office. For most individuals, home monitoring devices are more than adequate.

In fact, recent research published in the May 2006 issue of the *American Journal of Hypertension* shows that home monitoring is as effective and accurate as the far more expensive and inconvenient method of ABPM. This was the first study to directly compare the two methods. Please consider making a good investment in your heart health by purchasing a home monitoring device.

Below is the classification of blood pressure for adults eighteen years of age and older:

Classification	Systolic	Diastolic
Normal	Less than 120	Less than 80
Prehypertension	120–139	80–90
Stage 1 hypertension	140–159	90–99
Stage 2 hypertension	More than 160	More than 100

3

Different Blood Pressure Concerns for Different People

E levated blood pressure and hypertension know no ethnic or gender boundaries, afflicting men and women of all races all over the world. Yet every individual has special needs that must be taken into consideration.

Blood Pressure and Children

Cardiovascular disease in general and hypertension in particular begin in childhood. Studies indicate that children with elevated blood pressure levels are more prone to develop hypertension later in life, as early as in young adulthood. Percentages of youngsters with higher than normal blood pressure are increasing over time, perhaps owing to more sedentary behaviors and overweight. One estimate is that 30 percent of all overweight children have elevated blood pressure. Doctors are now seeing children as young as five years old with higher than normal blood pressure.

Normal blood pressure for children is, not surprisingly, lower than that for adults, and it gradually increases over the years. On average, systolic pressure will increase by 0.44 mm Hg annually for children between eight and twelve years old and by 2.90 between the ages of thirteen and seventeen. Diastolic blood pressure also gradually rises, by 0.33 from age eight to twelve and by 1.81 from thirteen to seventeen. Here's a chart to show typical blood pressure readings for youngsters between the ages of eight and seventeen.

Age	Blood Pressure in mm Hg (millimeters of mercury)
8	100/57
9	103/60
10	102/62
11	107/59
12	101/59
13	104/59
14	109/61
15	110/62
16	111/66
17	117/66

Especially in families with histories of cardiovascular disease and premature heart attacks and strokes, both blood pressure and cholesterol levels should be checked by the pediatrician or the family physician early in life. For reasons I personally cannot comprehend, there has been some controversy about doing so. It seems logical to me that a parent would want to know whether a son or a daughter has a greater than average potential to develop that disease later in life and to pay particular attention to encouraging a heart-healthy lifestyle in the entire family, complete with a heart-smart diet and plenty of physical activity. What parent would *not* want to give his or her child a future free of heart disease?

Good habits can be encouraged early in life and developed as easily as bad habits. My son, Ross, was six years old and Jenny was just three when I had my second bypass surgery. I did not want them to grow up to face the suffering I had undergone. A child's lifestyle is entirely dependent, especially very early in life, upon his or her parents. If fruit slices replace potato chips, kids will eat those healthier foods. If playing actively in the backyard and the park, with the whole family involved and perhaps some neighbor children as well, becomes the norm, less time will be spent in sedentary behaviors. We encourage our children to study hard at school and to do their homework. Why not be as interactive with their health as well?

If the pediatrician or the family physician doesn't automatically test for blood pressure during office visits, ask him or her to do so. Proper cuff size is critical to get accurate readings. One size does not fit all. A diagnosis of hypertension cannot properly be made at just one office visit. Readings must be high on three separate occasions at least one week apart. One estimate I read indicated that only about 10 percent of hypertensive children are diagnosed. This means that 90 percent of such kids are left to continue developing cardiovascular disease. To me that's unforgivable.

While being overweight plays the largest role in elevated blood pressure in childhood, other factors also enter the picture. Certainly, the physician will check for underlying disorders that can influence blood pressure. Since sleep disorders can affect blood pressure, be certain to mention any sleeping problems your child might be having. Smoking habits also play a role.

Swedish research shows that men born prematurely have a significantly greater risk of developing hypertension. Investigators studied more than three hundred thousand men born between 1973 and 1981 and who were drafted for military service between 1993 and 2001. Blood pressure readings of the young men born prematurely were proportionately elevated in a linear fashion, depending on the prematurity of the birth. Those born after less than twenty-nine weeks had almost twice the risk of high blood pressure; those born moderately preterm, from thirty-three to thirty-six weeks, had a 24 percent greater risk. The researchers recommend that children born prematurely have their blood pressure tested. While this study involved only young men, and the conclusions cannot be extrapolated to young women, it would appear wise to test all prematurely born children.

Hypertension is most typically silent in adults, with no symptoms, but that's not always true for children. More than half of children with untreated elevations in blood pressure experience frequent headaches, sleeping difficulties, daytime tiredness, and chest or other pains.

For most children with elevated blood pressure, treatment begins and ends with attaining a healthy weight and becoming more physically active. Children with other underlying causes of hypertension should be properly treated. Occasionally, a child's hypertension will be severe enough for the physician to consider prescribing a drug. Ultimately, that may be unavoidable. But why not attempt to lower blood pressure with one or more of the natural, harmless supplements I discuss in chapter 14? There's nothing to lose and everything to potentially gain.

Blood Pressure and African Americans

African Americans have one of the highest rates of hypertension in the world. Compared with whites, blacks are far more likely to have high blood pressure, to be overweight or obese, to live sedentary lifestyles and engage in less physical activity, to have diabetes, and to smoke cigarettes. That's a formula for disaster. Hypertension is the single largest factor for cardiovascular disease, stroke, kidney disease, and heart failure in African Americans. Similar combinations of traits can be found in other populations, such as Native Americans, who also have a higher incidence of hypertension. Ironically, in South Africa, white men have a higher prevalence of hypertension than black men do, although the situation is reversed in women there.

Results for such an explosive combination of risk factors are predictable. Estimates point to about 30 percent of non-Hispanic American white men and 24 percent of non-Hispanic white women having cardiovascular disease (CVD). For non-Hispanic blacks, those numbers leap to 41 percent of men and 40 percent of women with cardiovascular disease. Mexican Americans have statistics somewhere in the middle: about 29 percent of the men and 27 percent of the women have CVD.

The correlation between race and hypertension goes beyond medical and/or physiological explanations. It appears that racism itself has been shown to increase blood pressure in African Americans. That racism, according to researchers at Duke University in

North Carolina, doesn't even have to be overt; it can exert its influence just by being perceived. Doctors there measured twenty-four-hour ambulatory blood pressure, with monitors attached to subjects' bodies measuring blood pressure on a continuous basis throughout the day. Participants also filled out a report detailing episodes of racism and the resultant anger, but in order to live in a racist environment, those blacks had to repress their anger.

The major finding was that the differential between sleeping and waking blood pressure was less than average and certainly less than desirable. The greater the difference between night and day blood pressure, the better. Psychologically, African Americans were inhibiting their anger throughout the night in their subconscious thoughts, thus keeping blood pressure levels up.

The solution to the problem may well be more social than medical. In a project based at Johns Hopkins University in Baltimore, 309 urban African Americans participated in a program that included job referrals, career training, and housing assistance. At the end of a three-year period, the men who were part of the program had significantly better control of their hypertension than did those who did not participate.

Whether a reflection of the culture or of the pressures endured by lower socioeconomic groups, the use of illegal drugs, cigarette smoking, alcohol abuse, and dietary choices rich in saturated fats and sodium prevail in poor African American communities. One also finds a more defeatist attitude that would lead to rejection of suggestions for self-help health improvement.

Dietary concerns are critical among African Americans. Culturally ingrained eating habits are cherished or at least greatly enjoyed. Dishes are traditionally extremely high in salt. At the same time, blacks tend to be sodium sensitive. It's a matter of adding fuel to the fire. Thus the first drug of choice in this group most typically will be a diuretic to eliminate both stored fluids and sodium. Replacement of simultaneously lost potassium is essential, ideally by increasing potassium-rich foods and by encouraging the use of salt-replacement products that substitute potassium chloride for sodium chloride.

While there is no way to scientifically authenticate the following explanation of sodium sensitivity and hypertension in African Americans, the logic is intriguing. When Africans were loaded into ships bound for America for the slave trade, conditions were deplorable. Slaves were kept in the bowels of the ships where temperatures soared. Drinking water was insufficient, and dehydration led to numerous deaths. It has been speculated that the slaves with a genetic trait for retaining salt and water were able to survive. It is the genes of those surviving slaves that have been passed on through the generations in African Americans who are descendents of those poor souls.

Women, Hypertension, and Heart Disease

Traditionally, doctors have viewed heart disease as virtually the exclusive purview of men. Women presenting with identical symptoms would be diagnosed with something other than the heart disease that was, in fact, killing them. For decades, research dollars in cardiovascular disease were spent on studies that focused on men. Women were ignored. At best, there might be an afterthought in a journal publication that findings probably pertained to women as well as to men. In hindsight today, that was not always true.

The fact remains that cardiovascular disease is the number-one killer of both men and women. It is an equal opportunity agent of death. Yet despite years of efforts to educate women, surveys continue to show that women fear breast and ovarian cancers far more than they fear heart disease. One woman in eight will die of breast cancer; one in two will succumb to heart disease, dying of a heart attack or a stroke.

On levels beyond the obvious, women are very different from men. Their symptoms of a heart attack or angina pains will not be the dramatic crushing chest pain, the radiating pain from left shoulder down the arm, the feelings of indigestion, or the tightening of the jaw. Rather, women's symptoms might be a persistent and unexplained fatigue, feelings of lethargy, and emotional disturbances. Doctors have until recently viewed such symptoms chauvinistically and have prescribed tranquilizers and sleeping aids.

Though improvements have been made, a report from the American Heart Association on January 30, 2006, indicated that

- Women's chest pain is not taken as seriously as men's is.
- Women with stable chest pains are less likely than men are to be referred for diagnostic tests, receive bypass surgery or angioplasty, or be prescribed heart medications.
- Women are more likely than men are to be readmitted to the hospital after bypass surgery.
- Women are more likely than men are to have a worse outcome after coronary bypass surgery.

The intrinsic nature of women to put the needs of others, their family and friends, ahead of their own prevents them from seeking medical help at the first signs of cardiovascular disease. When women do present with such symptoms, doctors will still frequently either misdiagnose or dismiss them. Women have a higher rate of morbidity and mortality from heart attacks, strokes, angioplasties, and bypass surgeries, most likely because their disease has progressed far more than in men. For women of color, the statistics are much worse.

Hypertension takes a greater toll on women than on men. The risk of repeat heart attacks, strokes, and other cardiovascular events in women increases as blood pressure rises. In a prospective study of more than five thousand female health professionals with an average age of sixty-two, for each 10-point increase in systolic blood pressure a woman's cardiovascular disease risk increased by 9 percent. High blood pressure makes the heart work harder to pump blood throughout the body; that, in turn, causes the heart to enlarge and lose efficiency over time.

In the previous study, done at Brigham and Women's Hospital in Boston through the National Institutes of Health, researchers found an increased risk starting at a systolic pressure of 130. In the range of 130 to 139 systolic blood pressure, the risk was 28 percent greater than in women with blood pressure levels between 120 and 129. This is one more demonstration of the importance of paying attention to and lowering levels of what is now termed "prehypertension." Lifestyle modifications, especially in conjunction with new supplements, can effectively reduce prehypertension without the need for prescription drugs for women as well as for men.

The importance of one of those lifestyle modifications, increased physical activity, was showcased at the 2004 meeting of the American College of Cardiology. Fitness in women was shown to be the most important factor in assessing cardiac mortality risk. Every increase in fitness, measured on a treadmill, was associated with a 9 percent decrease in all-cause mortality and a 13 percent drop in cardiac mortality.

Here are some things for women to think about in terms of dealing with blood pressure and preventing or treating hypertension. Women have unique considerations.

Are you taking birth control pills? Researchers have determined that taking oral contraceptives is linked with higher blood pressure in some women, particularly if they're overweight. It's also a major consideration if you developed high blood pressure during pregnancy, have a family history of hypertension, or have kidney dysfunction. Taking birth control pills and smoking cigarettes is a dangerous combination. If you're thinking about starting on the pill, have your doctor measure your blood pressure and discuss these other conditions. If you're already taking the pill, have your blood pressure monitored regularly, preferably at home or in the doctor's office.

Hypertension can develop rapidly during the third trimester of pregnancy. Untreated, it can pose a danger to both mother and child. So-called gestational hypertension commonly disappears after pregnancy but not always. And if your blood pressure was elevated prior to pregnancy it's particularly important to monitor it on a regular basis.

Without making any moral judgments, it is a fact that women are more prone to gain weight as they age and are more likely to become obese. Both overweight and obesity greatly increase the risk of elevated blood pressure and hypertension.

Blood pressure tends to rise as both women and men age, but the risk of developing hypertension increases significantly following menopause.

Whether it's true that women eventually become their mothers, if your mother had high blood pressure, your odds of developing the disease increase substantially. That's also true for diabetes. If you have those diseases in your family history, forewarned should be forearmed.

Blood Pressure and Older Men and Women

Throughout the Western world, as well as in rapidly developing nations, the percentage of older men and women is rapidly increasing. In lockstep with advancing age, blood pressure rises. Data from the internationally renowned Framingham study show that 27 percent of people younger than age sixty have blood pressure readings higher than 140/90 and 20 percent have frank hypertension with measurements of 160/100. That's pretty bad. But among people older than eighty, nearly 75 percent are hypertensive (higher than 140/90) and 60 percent are at 160/100 or higher. Only 7 percent of the oldest group studied, those over eighty, had normal blood pressure.

Unfortunately, the percentage of hypertensive older men and women being treated is lower than doctors would like to see. And of those receiving treatment, the number of older people achieving their blood pressure goals is far from desirable.

Many doctors still believe that aggressively treating older patients is unproductive. They maintain that few of them are willing to go along with medical advice. And some doctors have said to me in private conversations that they don't want to ask older men and women to change their lifestyles, giving up some of their favorite foods and exercising more than they've done in perhaps decades. After all, such doctors say, those men and women don't have that many years left anyway, and they may as well enjoy all their simple pleasures. What a pile of condescending crap!

It has been my distinct pleasure to work with a number of organizations of older men and women, doing presentations for church groups, hospitals, self-help groups, and retirement communities. I started doing so shortly after my first book was published in 1987, and I've done it ever since. I must say that of all the audiences I address, none is more attentive and open to suggestions. I love it when I drive into retirement villages and see men and women in their sweatshirts and sweatpants briskly walking, arms pumping back and forth, along established paths.

I think those doctors I previously referred to have lost perspective. Many older men and women are accurately described as "Golden Agers." They've worked hard all their lives, raised their children, and now are enjoying their earthly rewards, in no particular hurry to seek their eternal rewards. They love their grandchildren and enjoy spoiling them in spite of their sons' and daughters' disapproval. They look forward to vacations and holidays, whether their financial circumstances allow for cruises on luxury ships in the Mediterranean Sea or trips in buses to see the autumnal color changes in the leaves of trees. They take pleasure in gathering in community halls for bingo games and bridge tournaments or to hear a lecture from an author such as myself.

I leave those occasions with a huge smile on my face and feel that I've learned far more than I've taught. What I've learned is that no matter how old one gets, life is enjoyed more completely in good health and that health and vitality are worth working for. Those senior citizens are indeed willing to change their dietary habits—at least reasonably so. They'll engage in physical activity, especially when such activity can be fun, such as gardening or walking with friends. Despite what many doctors believe, older patients are willing to take their medications—when they understand what those meds do, how they work, and what side effects, if any, might be expected. After all, they might say about such side effects, life has its trade-offs.

Indeed, some of the side effects that might keep younger men and women from being compliant with their prescriptions become less troublesome for older people. If a pill causes one to become a bit tired in the middle of the day, it might be nice to take a nap! If a diuretic pill means more trips to the bathroom, that's okay, too.

One of the potential added benefits of treating and controlling blood pressure in older patients is a reduced risk of dementia. Investigators at the National Institute of Aging in Bethesda, Maryland, have observed that the longer a person is treated for hypertension—that is to say, the faster one begins to control blood pressure—the lower the dementia risk becomes. These findings appear to dismiss previous concerns that lowering blood pressure might have a negative effect on cognitive function. Quite the opposite seems to be true. Compared to people who were never treated for hypertension, patients in the study who had been treated for twelve years or more had 60 percent less dementia risk than people who had never been treated.

Ultimately, your physician will make the decision as to which drug or drugs might be best for you, at least to start with. If you have a good relationship with him or her—as you should have, for heaven's sake—you can experiment until you find the winning combination.

Older individuals often have structural and functional damage to the aorta, the large artery leading out from the heart, that causes increased stiffness and resultant increased blood pressure. Some studies have shown that calcium channel blockers and diuretics are drug classes that are particularly useful in treating older patients' hypertension; perhaps that's because those drugs provide greater reductions in aortic pressures than do other drugs such as beta blockers. Other studies have come up with completely opposite conclusions. Work with your doctor as a functional doctor-patient team.

Read the chapter on drugs later in the book. It'll be good for you to more completely understand how they work. You'll impress your physician! And consider taking one or more of the supplements that can improve arterial health and reduce blood pressure naturally. Even if those supplements can't do the job on their own, and in older individuals they're less likely to do so, they can help to reduce needed drug dosages and improve the flexibility and elasticity of your arteries. That's a good thing.

As I come to the end of writing this chapter, I'm filled with a lot of thoughts. Memories of establishing heart-healthy habits in my children, Ross and Jenny, and happiness that both of them have carried those habits into young adulthood. Greater realization of the problems of ethnic groups less fortunate than I. The need to be supportive of my wife's special needs. And a flood of amazement that when I began doing those presentations at churches, hospitals, and retirement villages, I was considered a youngster in my middle forties and now I'm approaching my own Golden Age. Yet two things have definitely not changed: first, the burning desire to share helpful health information with others and second, my own willingness to work as hard as ever to stay healthy myself, to forego those fatty but tasty dessert temptations, and to exercise even when my muscles and bones complain in their inimitable achy language. Because life indeed is worth living to the fullest, and the only way to do that is to stay as healthy as possible. The arthritis in my hands and the pain in my back from degenerative disks that come with being in my sixties won't hold me down!

4

Blood Pressure and Diabetes

Most doctors I spoke with while I did research for this book said virtually the same thing: "I consider every diabetic patient to be a heart patient." That was confirmed by a 2002 survey done by the American Diabetes Association (ADA) and the American College of Cardiology (ACC). More than 90 percent of physicians surveyed reported that men and women with diabetes are "very likely" or "extremely likely" to have a cardiovascular event.

There's a good reason all those physicians feel that way. Fully 65 percent of diabetic men and women will die from a heart attack or a stroke. Yet diabetic patients are not sufficiently conscious of their risk. In another survey done by the ADA and the ACC that same year, 68 percent of diabetics reported that they were not aware of their increased risk for heart disease and stroke. Indeed, those cardiovascular events strike diabetics more than twice as often as they do other people.

Prehypertension poses particular hazards for diabetic men and women, as found in a study at the University of Oklahoma Health Sciences Center. Doctors there investigated prehypertension in 2,629 subjects taking part in the Strong Heart Study. Many within that group—42 percent—had diabetes. At the outset, participants had normal blood pressure and were free of heart disease. They were followed for twelve years, during which time 389 people suffered a heart event.

Researchers examined the data and found that compared with nondiabetic individuals with normal blood pressure, those with diabetes and prehypertension had nearly four times the risk of experiencing a cardiovascular incident such as a heart attack or a stroke. Those with diabetes alone had 2.9 times the average risk and those with prehypertension alone had 1.8 times the average risk. The take-home message here is obvious: if you have both diabetes and prehypertension you are at greatly increased risk.

A diagnosis of diabetes in an adult presents the same degree of risk as someone who has already had a heart attack. Cardiovascular complications happen at earlier ages and often result in premature death. People with diabetes are five times more likely to suffer strokes and, after the first stroke, are two to four times more likely to have a second one.

While cardiovascular disease statistics seem to be improving for the general population, those gains are not shared by diabetics. Quite to the contrary. Deaths from heart disease in women with diabetes have increased by 23 percent over the past thirty years, while there has been a 27 percent *decrease* in women without diabetes. Deaths for diabetic men have increased by 13 percent, but men without diabetes have enjoyed a 36 percent decrease.

That's why it is absolutely essential that men and women with diabetes learn and practice their ABCs. "A" stands for hemoglobin A1C, typically stated simply as A1C. This is a measurement of average glucose, blood sugar, levels over a two- to three-month period. Have that test done at least twice a year; you'll want the results to be less than 7 percent. "B" represents blood pressure. We'll discuss that in detail in this chapter; your target should be less than 130/80 mm Hg, the definition of hypertension for diabetic individuals, as compared with 140/80 for people without the disease. Of course, the lower the better. And "C" stands for cholesterol, especially the "bad" LDL cholesterol. Yours should be less than 100 mg/dl—as low as possible. You'll want to pay particular attention to chapter 11.

Hypertension: Even More Important in Diabetes Care

Hypertension is pervasive in people with diabetes. In the United States, the Third National Health and Nutrition Survey (NHANES) found that 71 percent of all diabetic men and women had hypertension. Twenty-nine percent of them were unaware that they had elevated blood pressure. Forty-three percent were untreated. Even diabetics being treated had a blood pressure of more than 140/90. Only 12 percent in treatment had reached the goal of less than 130/80.

Diabetic men and women have an increased likelihood of developing prehypertension, if not full-blown hypertension. Prehypertension puts everyone, and especially diabetics, at greater risk of developing cardiovascular disease and predicts that if left uncontrolled, hypertension will follow. The risk of developing cardiovascular disease for diabetic individuals is 3.60 times as great as that for nondiabetic men and women with normal blood pressure. That's a huge differential in risk!

The good news, after all those dreadful statistics that I hated to report but felt I had to give you, is that diabetes in general and hypertension in particular can be controlled, and complications and risks can be greatly reduced. The first step must be to make the commitment to yourself and to the people you love and who love you.

My wife, Dawn, worked with a fellow high school teacher who was only in her early thirties but was obese. The woman actually requested that she be assigned no classes on the second floor because she was unable to walk up the stairs and there was no elevator. She ate huge amounts of food and was completely sedentary. One day she told Dawn that her doctor had diagnosed her as having diabetes. Her response was startling; she said that she'd expected to get the disease since her mother and grandmother both had it, but she hadn't expected to develop diabetes so soon. Yet even after that diagnosis the woman did nothing to lose weight or to become more active.

A friend of mine, who had already suffered a massive heart attack, was told by his physician that if he did not control his diabetes, he not only was under great risk of having a second attack but could also expect lower limb amputations and kidney failure requiring dialysis. Surely, you would think, that got his attention. No, he has now lost a few toes and walks with a cane, he undergoes dialysis that leaves him exhausted twice a week, and he can no longer work.

Only you can make the commitment. I can only hope that since you're now reading this book, you're open to suggestions that can save your life and make it a lot more enjoyable.

Controlling Blood Pressure and Diabetes

In many ways, you have a two-for-the-price-of-one situation. The same lifestyle modifications detailed throughout this book will help to control both diabetes and high blood pressure. In fact, the guidelines for the initial treatment of diabetics with a blood pressure reading of 130–139/80–89 call for a three-month trial of nondrug treatment prior to starting a patient on antihypertensive drugs.

Those modifications include weight loss, increased physical activity, smoking cessation, moderation of alcohol consumption, and restricted sodium intake. All are detailed in this book. The ADA and the ACC note in a publication for physicians that weight loss can reduce blood pressure, even without changing sodium, and that losing just 2.2 pounds (1 kilogram) results, on average, in a decrease of 1 blood pressure point. How much weight should you lose? Only you can give an honest answer to that question. Whatever the number of pounds, each one lost can lower your blood pressure. That can be very significant. Increasing your physical activity to an average of thirty to forty-five minutes a day on most days of the week, with a brisk walk as an example, can further lower your blood pressure.

The wonderful thing is that men and women who lose a sufficient amount of weight and who become physically active can actually "cure" not only their elevated blood pressure but also diabetes itself. Daily measurements of glucose and periodic tests of A1C can show a return to normal levels. The diagnosis of diabetes is tentatively made when blood sugar rises above 126. A definitive diagnosis is established by a reading of more than 7 percent on the A1C test. Conversely, when blood sugar levels fall below 126 and A1C is less than 7 percent, a person's diabetes is "cured." I use the quotation marks here because once diabetes is established, the person must be vigilant on a lifelong basis to keep glucose and A1C counts normal, lest diabetes return. But, for all practical purposes, your diabetes would be cured, without the quotation marks. This means that the risk of developing cardiovascular disease and other complications of diabetes, including potential kidney damage, blindness, and amputations, is greatly reduced. Isn't that worth working for?

Nearly all physicians feel that the vast majority of diabetic patients will require more than one drug, often as many as three, to control hypertension. Most doctors will begin with an ACE inhibitor (see chapter 16) and will add other drugs as needed. Those drugs, of course, come with a raft of potential side effects, so it would be well worth your while to do your level best to get your blood pressure down without needing them. Your doctor won't be disappointed. Trust me when I say that more doctors would give the lifestyle modifications more credence and be in less of a hurry to reach for the prescription pad if they felt that their patients would do their utmost to achieve the desired goals through weight loss, exercise, stress management, and so forth. Sadly, most patients do not, and physicians have come to expect that failure. Prove your doctor wrong!

While working hard to lose weight and increase physical activity, you'll also want to use the special weapons described in chapter 14. All those supplements have been shown to increase levels of nitric oxide, as I explain, a gas that keeps arteries flexible, elastic, and capable of dilation to allow for increased blood flow as needed. They all have been shown to lower blood pressure. It's the pressure of blood flow against less flexible and elastic arteries that we know as hypertension.

In reading that chapter, you'll want to pay particular attention to the supplement Pycnogenol, derived from French maritime pine trees. Pycnogenol has been seen to increase nitric oxide production within the arteries.

Dr. Ximing Liu explained his reason for researching the potential of Pycnogenol by citing patients who no longer needed insulin to treat their type 2 diabetes. He and his associates wanted to determine whether Pycnogenol has a glucose-lowering effect. They recruited eighteen men and twenty-two women who were outpatients at their hospital. Those subjects ranged in age from twenty-eight to sixty-four and were of normal weight, overweight, or obese. Patients were given 50, 100, 200, and 300 mg doses of Pycnogenol in three-week intervals. Every three weeks glucose levels (both fasting and after a meal), A1C, and insulin were measured. The researchers reported a linear, dose-dependent reduction in glucose levels when patients took up to 200 mg of Pycnogenol. A 300 mg dose provided no further benefit. Both fasting glucose and measurements following meals were significantly lower.

A1C levels fell continuously from 8.02 ± 1.04 to 7.37 ± 1.09. Improvement was noted from nine to twelve weeks with 200 or 300 mg of Pycnogenol. There was no difference in insulin levels, indicating that beneficial changes did not owe to increased insulin secretion.

The investigators did a follow-up study with seventy-seven type 2 diabetic patients who took a glucose-lowering medication (hypoglycemic agent). Once again, Pycnogenol significantly lowered blood glucose.

Although no one knows the exact mode of action by which Pycnogenol lowers blood glucose levels in diabetic patients, researchers have speculated that the powerful antioxidant supplement seems to overcome the blocked glucose uptake by cells in the body. Interestingly, in studies with diabetic rats, Pycnogenol significantly lowered blood glucose, while there was no such response in normal rats.

Magnesium, Metabolic Syndrome, Diabetes, and Hypertension

As I explain in chapter 9, it may be more important to increase and thus balance levels of minerals in the body (electrolytes), including magnesium, calcium, and potassium, than it is to reduce the mineral sodium in our diets. As I titled that chapter, it's an electrolyte balancing act. It appears that magnesium may play a role in diabetes as well.

Researchers at Northwestern University in Chicago noted that previous studies indicated that magnesium is inversely related to the risk of developing hypertension and type 2 diabetes; that is to say, the more magnesium in the diet, the less chance of those diseases developing. So they looked at the relationship between magnesium intake and a precursor of diabetes called the metabolic syndrome, which includes high blood pressure, overweight, inefficiency of insulin termed *insulin resistance*, high levels of triglycerides, and lower than desired levels of the protective HDL cholesterol. Magnesium has also been observed to lower triglycerides and increase HDL.

For fifteen years, the study tracked 4,637 men who were eighteen to thirty years old at the start of the project. During that time, there were 608 cases of metabolic syndrome. Magnesium intake was inversely associated with the incidence of that syndrome. That, in turn, can potentially reduce the future incidence of diabetes.

That research was reported only in 2006. There have been no studies yet as to whether increasing magnesium consumption in the diet and taking supplements will improve diabetes. That said, the Northwestern investigators noted that "Experimental data suggest that magnesium may directly regulate cellular glucose metabolism," and that "magnesium intake may improve insulin sensitivity." Both of those functions of this mineral would be enormously important for the diabetic patient. The recommended daily intake is 500 mg.

I mentioned my friend who ignored both his doctor's advice and my urging to control his diabetes. I won't be surprised when I get the phone call that he has passed away. What a terrible waste. And in the meantime, the quality of his life is impaired.

I'll end this chapter with one more set of statistics, not to scare you but rather to encourage you to make your best possible effort to control both your diabetes and your hypertension. By all means, try the lifestyle modifications, including diet and exercise, and give the supplements a chance. But if they don't take you all the way to a solid reduction of hypertension, I urge you to work with your physician to find the prescription medications that can save your life. Yes, those drugs can be associated with side effects. But by working with your doctor you can find one or more that will give you the blood pressure reduction you need while minimizing the adverse side effects.

So now, here are the final diabetes statistics from the Centers for Disease Control and Prevention in the United States, which I quote directly from the report in the *Journal of the American Medical Association*: "If an individual is diagnosed at age 40 years, men will lose 11.6 life-years and 18.6 quality-adjusted life-years and women will lose 14.3 life-years and 22.0 quality-adjusted life-years." Those extra years of life and quality of life are well worth working for.

PART TWO

The Blood Pressure Cure Program

5

Weight and Blood Pressure

Men and women are getting fatter and fatter, and we're paying the price for those supersize meals with an increased risk of developing high blood pressure, diabetes, heart attacks, and strokes. The scariest statistic I've read is that today's youngsters, who are heavier and more sedentary than ever, will be the first generation with a life expectancy *shorter* than that of their parents.

When it comes to weight, we are definitely living in a global community. Nearly two-thirds of all American men and women are overweight or obese. In Canada, 40.6 percent of women and 58 percent of men are overweight or obese. Statistics from the Australian Society for the Study of Obesity indicate that more than half of all Australian women and two-thirds of men share that dubious distinction. In the United Kingdom, 40 percent of men and 33 percent of women are overweight and 20 percent are obese. A surgeon in the Netherlands commented that he had to put two operating tables together to operate on one heavy patient. Some patients there barely fit into scanning machines.

As people gain weight, their risk of developing hypertension grows along with them. Conversely, data show that even moderate weight loss reduces that risk. One study's investigators followed 623 middle-aged disease-free adults, thirty to forty-nine years old, and 605 older adults, ages fifty to sixty-five. People who lost fifteen pounds or more reduced their long-term risk of developing hypertension by 21 percent, while older adults losing that much weight enjoyed a 29 percent drop in risk.

Weight gain and blood pressure are in lockstep. The more overweight a person becomes, the higher his or her blood pressure will likely go. Happily, though, the more weight an overweight individual manages to lose, the better his or her blood pressure control will be. Losing weight is, in fact, one of the most solidly documented lifestyle modifications shown to improve blood pressure.

Cutting-edge research for the past several years has focused on the importance of maintaining the health of the endothelium, the lining of the inside of the artery. A healthy endothelium does not develop atherosclerosis as much as an unhealthy, inflamed arterial lining. Hence there have been dozens of papers published in the medical literature concluding that inflammation is a major risk factor or at least a risk marker for heart disease. Happily, one of the best ways to reduce inflammation is with weight loss.

Writing in the January 8, 2007, issue of the *Archives of Internal Medicine*, doctors at Johns Hopkins University in Baltimore found that weight loss, whether through dieting, exercise, or even surgery, dramatically lowered inflammation as measured by C-reactive protein, commonly termed CRP. The more weight lost, the more substantial the CRP improvements. Dr. Elizabeth Selvin pointed out that fat cells are directly involved in the production of CRP and other inflammatory markers of heart disease risk.

The statistical links between weight and cardiovascular disease are flat-out scary. One of the most definitive studies began in 1967. Data were collected until 2002. During those years, subjects were classified as normal weight, overweight, or obese. The risk of being hospitalized for heart problems quadrupled in men and women after age sixty-five in the obese group. Obese individuals were also more likely to die from heart attacks and strokes than thinner persons were.

Classifying Weight and Risk

We all have our ways of knowing when we're overweight. Our clothes don't fit the way they used to. We loosen our belts a notch. Stepping on the bathroom scales isn't something we really want to do. Simple acts of movement such as getting out of a chair, much less walking up a flight of stairs, become increasingly difficult.

Yet medical researchers have more precise methods to classify overweight and obesity. One of the most common classification systems is called the body-mass index or BMI. This measurement system long ago replaced old insurance tables. BMI is a single number that represents weight and height without regard to age or gender. BMI is calculated by dividing your height in inches squared (multiplied by itself) into your weight in pounds multiplied by the number 703.

$$BMI = \frac{(\text{weight in pounds} \times 703)}{\text{height in inches}^2}$$

In the metric system, that would be your weight in kilograms divided by your height in meters squared. But don't worry about doing the math. I've done that for some representative heights and weights in the following table, taken from the World Health Organization (WHO), providing BMIs for a range of heights and weights.

A BMI of 24 or less is considered healthy and normal. A BMI of 25, 26, or 27 would indicate overweight. And a BMI of 30 or more classifies a person as being obese.

BODY-MASS INDEX SCALE

Height	Weight (lb.)				
5 ft. 1 in.	127	132	137	143	158
5 ft. 2 in.	131	136	142	147	164
5 ft. 3 in.	135	141	146	152	169
5 ft. 4 in.	140	145	151	157	174
5 ft. 5 in.	144	150	156	162	180
5 ft. 6 in.	148	155	161	167	186
5 ft. 7 in.	153	159	166	172	191
5 ft. 8 in.	158	164	171	177	197
5 ft. 9 in.	162	169	176	182	203
5 ft. 10 in.	167	174	181	188	207
5 ft. 11 in.	172	179	186	193	215
6 ft.	177	184	191	199	221
6 ft. 1 in.	182	189	197	204	227
BMI	24	25	26	27	30

There's one major problem with the BMI system. What about an athletic man or woman? Muscle weighs more than fat tissue. A football player who stands 6 feet 1 inch and weighs 204 pounds may be solid muscle with very little fat. He would scarcely be thought of as overweight, despite a BMI of 27 that would put him into that classification. A bodybuilder might even weigh 227 at that same height, but he wouldn't be called obese.

Some authorities believe that changing the standard from BMI to waist-to-hip ratio would improve the accuracy of cardiovascular risk determinations. That was the conclusion of the INTER-HEART study involving more than twenty-seven thousand participants from fifty-two countries.

Others would prefer a simple measurement of waist circumference (WC) to determine weight-related health risk. Stratification for men would be a WC less than 38 inches, from 38 to 42 inches, and more than 42 inches for normal, overweight, and obese. For women it would be a WC less than 33 inches, from 33 to 36 inches, and more than 36 inches.

I think the best approach was proposed by Canadian researchers who presented a spectrum of studies and convincingly argued for combining both BMI and WC to calculate risk. Take a look at the BMI table and see whether your height and weight would classify you as normal weight, overweight, or obese. Then look at your waist circumference. Put the two together and you've got a pretty good idea of your personal risk.

Of course, I hope that you fall into the normal weight category. But if you do, you probably wouldn't be reading this chapter other than perhaps out of curiosity.

Which Diet Is Best?

Ultimately, the best diet is the one you'll stick with long enough not only to lose weight but also to change and improve your eating habits. It will do no good to lose those extra pounds only to gain them right back along with a few more; actually, that sort of yo-yo dieting harms your body.

While there have been dozens of diet books, many of which reached the best-seller list, all of them fall into one category or another. Perhaps you've tried one or more of those diets.

- **Gimmick diets** advise that you concentrate on one or another food (the grapefruit or cabbage soup diets), never combine foods of different types at one time (Fit for Life and others), combine foods in a very specified manner (the Zone diet and others), alternate certain foods throughout the week, splurge after "being good" for a few days, or do some sort of fasting. The next time you might be tempted to try one of those fad diets, ask yourself whether you could really imagine eating that way for the rest of your life.
- **Low-carb diets** promise that you can eat all the rich foods you want, from beef to bacon to butter, but must eliminate most carbohydrate-containing foods. The Atkins diet is currently the most famous of these, although they have been around for decades in one incarnation or another. As mouth-watering as this approach might sound at the start, no matter how much you love bacon and eggs pretty soon you'll be lusting for a slice of toast and marmalade and a glass of orange juice to go with that breakfast. Rapid weight loss comes from water loss. And studies have shown that most low-carb dieters usually abandon the program after no more than six months.
- **Low-fat diets** tempt dieters—and potential book buyers—with the idea that one can eat all one wants and still lose weight. Theoretically, that's true since low-fat foods typically are bulky and filling. But, as with the low-carb diets, these regimens get boring mighty fast, especially if they're vegetarian diets.

Researchers at Tufts University in Boston decided to put a number of diets to the test. They recruited 160 overweight or obese adults with an average BMI of 35 in a range of 27 to 42. Subjects were put on the Atkins low-carb diet, the Zone diet of combined food specifications, the Ornish ultra-low-fat near-vegetarian diet, or the Weight Watchers balanced diet that restricts calories. They each were given the book that spelled out the particular diet, with no additional instruction or guidance. Participants were asked to stick with the diet for one year, but only 53 percent stuck with Atkins, 65 percent followed through with the Zone diet, 65 percent with Weight Watchers, and 50 percent with Ornish.

Weight loss was just about the same at the end of the year for all programs, with average reductions of 4.6 pounds for Atkins, 7.0 for the Zone, 6.6 for Weight Watchers, and 7.3 for Ornish. Not surprisingly, with such small weight losses, blood pressure measurements were virtually unchanged. As the authors of the study wrote, "Overall dietary adherence rates were low, although increased adherence was associated with greater weight loss and cardiac risk factor reductions for each diet group."

The problem with all those diets, as is true with any diet, is that for virtually everyone, going on a diet means going off that diet. The only approach that really works is to change one's lifestyle enough to reduce the number of calories taken in as food and to increase the amount of calories burned through physical activity. In other words, you need to go on the "No-Fad Diet," as Dr. Robert Eckel called it in his editorial accompanying the article that compared the four diets mentioned above.

The diet that works for one person won't necessarily work for you. If you absolutely love ice cream, a diet that forbids it is bound to fail. If a dinner isn't complete without a piece of bread and a glass of wine, your diet must include them both. Simply enough, you need your very own personal "Diet for the Rest of Your Life."

In the Gordian knot legend, people tried and tried to figure out a way to unravel an intricately woven knot. He who did so would be named king. Finally, Alexander the Great simply walked up and sliced through the knot with a single stroke of his sword. Ultimately, weight control can be likened to that Gordian knot. We can slice through all the complications and gimmicks very simply to reveal the essential knowledge we need to lose weight, maintain that weight loss, and remain healthy while lowering blood pressure. There are certain foods we want to eat a lot of and others we should limit. No radical gimmickry here, just straightforward logic—like cutting through that knot.

Foods to emphasize provide a lot of nutrients as well as fiber and protective plant substances called polyphenols. These include fruits, vegetables, and whole-grain breads and cereals. To those, add at least weekly two servings, preferably three or even four, of fish and seafood, especially the fatty fish rich in omega-3 fatty acids that are so good for our hearts. But there's no reason to eliminate red meat; just choose the leanest cuts of beef, pork, lamb, and veal. Try to have two or three daily servings of nonfat or low-fat dairy foods; not just milk but also yogurt and cheese for their calcium and other nutrients. Enjoy nuts in moderation as a healthy snack and lots of dishes made from dried beans and peas that provide soluble fiber to lower cholesterol and improve blood pressure. For weight-management purposes, go easy on the oils, which, while healthy, concentrate 120 calories per tablespoon.

Foods to limit or even avoid, at least during your weight-loss efforts, are those that provide little or no nutritional value but a lot of empty calories. In restaurants, ask the server not to bring a bread-basket. Avoid that temptation entirely. And at home limit white bread. Each slice you give up knocks at least 100 calories from your daily intake. The same goes for pasta and rice; sure, they're delicious, but they offer nothing but calories. Needless to say, people trying to lose weight should virtually eliminate cake, candies, cookies, and other sweets. At the very least, opt for the smallest portions of high-cal treats. After dinner in the evening a steaming mug of hot cocoa made with a calorie-free sweetener such as Splenda (sucralose) is relaxing, comforting, and satisfying without the calories.

Really and truly, that's all the nutrition advice, in a nutshell, you need to very successfully lose weight and ultimately maintain a healthy weight and blood pressure for the rest of your life. And it'll be a longer, more enjoyable life.

Start Writing Your Own Diet Book

Actually, I mean that subhead quite literally. The best way to begin a successful weight loss, and ultimately lifelong weight control, pro-gram is to critically analyze what you're eating and drinking, to learn which foods and beverages are keeping you overweight. I suggest that you start writing a daily diary or journal.

Record everything, and I do mean everything, you eat and drink and when you consume those foods and beverages. The closer you get to being your own personal researcher, the better. Don't just jot down that you "had some soda in the afternoon." Specify what kind of soda and how much you drank. Invest in a kitchen scale you can use to weigh those servings of food. Is it an 8-ounce glass of soda or a quart? Was it a 4-ounce steak or a pound? Did you snack on a few nuts or the entire can? Start paying attention to the calories in the foods you eat. Be totally honest with yourself.

Keep that food and beverage log for a full week, eating as you normally do and not trying to get a jump-start on your diet or fooling yourself. I hope you're not the sort of person who cheats at solitaire!

After a week of scrupulous note taking, read and critique your eating and drinking habits. Look at that journal as though it were written by someone else. Put yourself into the role of dietitian. Where would it be fairly painless to cut back on serving sizes? A glass of red wine with a small lean steak for dinner protects against cardiovascular disease in a delicious way. But a full bottle washing down a one-pound chunk of well-marbled beef may be a bit excessive, don't you agree? What foods provide lots of calories with little or no nutrient value? When are you snacking? While watching TV in the evening after a stressful day?

What are the changes you're willing to make and which eating habits would you fight to the death for? Simply must have that dish of ice cream in the evening? Not a problem. But could you switch to a low-fat brand, reduce the serving size by about half, and top the dish off with some fresh berries? Could you make that slice of toast in the morning whole-grain and spread it with a bit of trans fat–free tub margarine and a dab of low-cal preserves? If watching TV in the living room or the family room downstairs prompts you to gorge on snacks, could you go upstairs and read a book instead, thus breaking the Pavlovian connection? Or could you plan in advance to have snacks that won't expand your waistline? Perhaps a platter of freshly sliced oranges and apples? Or some popcorn or pretzels?

Only you can make the choices you'll be able to live with. Don't try to change everything at once. Little things can truly mean a lot. I'm always reminded when I write or speak about such things of the day my late father-in-law, Ben, told the family he was going to shed the twelve-pound spare tire around his waist by not putting sugar in his coffee. Everyone laughed, thinking that such an insignificant thing couldn't possibly make a difference, especially a twelve-pound difference.

But think about the numbers. One teaspoon of sugar has 16 calories. Ben added three spoons to his coffee and drank five cups daily. Multiply 16 times three teaspoons and then multiply those 48 calories by five cups for a total of 240 calories a day, 7,200 calories a month. That number of calories yields 2 pounds of weight loss or gain. In six months, Ben lost those 12 pounds without doing anything else!

Preemptive Snacking

No matter what sort of diet you follow in order to lose weight, and I'll discuss those options in the coming pages, I have a tip that's certain to help. It all began with research done in the 1960s at Michigan State University. The study was very simple, especially when compared with the complex projects of today. Women who wanted to lose weight were given only one instruction: twenty to thirty minutes before meals, they were to eat a slice of bread. Participants in the study who followed that advice lost weight in a very satisfying manner.

How and why did that simple change work? As we eat, food is converted to blood sugar, glucose, that enters the bloodstream to provide energy for the body. It takes about twenty minutes for sensors in the brain to pick up the fact that blood sugar levels have risen and that there isn't a need for more food. As those glucose levels rise, we're no longer hungry. The problem is that when we're really hungry and start to eat, we don't give the body and the brain time to recognize that sugar levels have gone up. We shouldn't be hungry any longer, but we continue to eat.

By eating that slice of bread twenty to thirty minutes before lunch and dinner, women in the MSU study caused their blood sugar levels to rise before they sat down to eat the meal. When they did so, they weren't as hungry and didn't eat as much as they would have otherwise. They lost weight.

I put this into practice when my children were little. I was trying to establish a heart-healthy lifestyle to protect them from heart disease later in life. That meant limiting the cake, cookies, ice cream, pizza, and so forth. So when they were invited to birthday parties or elsewhere, about twenty minutes before we were to leave the house I'd ask whether they were hungry. Of course, little kids are always hungry! So I'd give them a healthy snack of some sliced fruit, a small sandwich, a cup of soup, or something like that. When they got to the party, they weren't ravenous and therefore ate a lot less of the fatty foods than they would have otherwise.

Many individuals have practiced this "preemptive snacking" without realizing it. Whoever is preparing the evening's meal will frequently taste foods while cooking. While peeling the carrots, most of us will eat one or two. When setting out the bread, both my wife and I tend to break off the heel and eat it. Do that a few times and blood sugar begins to rise and one isn't as hungry when dinner is served to the rest of the family.

Make preemptive snacking part of your lifestyle. Start with breakfast. If you're not in a hurry to get out of the house, drink your glass of juice or have a slice of toast with the first cup of coffee twenty to thirty minutes before sitting down to the full meal. If you've "brown-bagged it" for lunch at work, you won't overeat since there'll be only a limited amount of food in that bag. But if you're heading out for lunch, remember to have that snack before you leave.

Ultimately, the ideal would be to never get very hungry. Make sure to have another healthy snack midafternoon. This doesn't mean the typical doughnut and coffee. Instead, make it a handful of nuts or dried fruit or perhaps a granola bar.

The evening meal offers the most temptation to overeat. Rather than waiting for dinner to be served, whether you're cooking it or not, get into the healthy habit of eating a rather substantial snack well before dinner. I personally enjoy some herring on whole-grain crackers. Or I might have a cup of yogurt. I keep bite-size precut vegetables—the French call this crudités—in the refrigerator to munch on while watching the evening news as my wife prepares dinner or while I prepare the dinner if it's my turn to cook.

Give preemptive snacking a try for a couple of weeks and see if that doesn't make you eat less at major meals. To be most successful, keep a supply of healthy snacks on hand so that they're readily available.

Avoid Stress Eating

I love living in this modern age with all of its wonderful advances and advantages, but stress is part and parcel of life for most of us. The higher the level of stress during the day, the more likely we'll use food in the evening as a coping mechanism. We eat continuously not because we're hungry but simply as a nervous instinct. I suppose it's a better habit than self-medicating into anesthesia with booze, but it's still not very healthy.

The emphasis in that last sentence should be on the word *habit*. We get into a deeply embedded habit of nonstop eating in the evening, especially when watching television or a DVD. Fortunately, there are a few ways to deal with that bad habit.

The easiest thing is to accept the habit and simply try to modify it a bit. Think about your own evening snacking. If you're like most people, you head for the refrigerator or the pantry and grab the first food you see. If the food happens to be salty potato chips, that's what you'll eat, and very likely you'll devour the entire bag. Instead of serving yourself a small dish of ice cream, you'll take the tub out and dig in with a spoon, sometimes until there's no more ice cream left.

Let's modify those habits. What if those chips aren't in the pantry at all, and instead you find some nuts in their shells? Put a handful or two in a bowl along with a nut cracker and dig out the nut meats in front of the TV. The idea is to keep your hands busy shelling the nuts rather than eating mixed nuts out of a can.

Make your own popcorn from scratch rather than popping the microwaveable types that are loaded with trans-fatty acids. The aromas that fill the house are wonderful and put you into a much more relaxed mode.

An alternative that I strongly prefer is making a steaming cup of hot cocoa. Low in fat and calories, that cup of cocoa relaxes the mind and can help to lower blood pressure, thanks to its polyphenol content. See the recipe section at the end of the book for preparation tips. I personally find that I get a much better night's sleep after drinking a mug of cocoa.

As a complete alternative to snacking, keep one of those squeezable rubber balls or worry beads or something else nearby to occupy your hands instead of eating. Try putting a couple of lightweight dumbbells next to the couch or the chair and keep busy doing some exercise.

Or try to break the conditioned-response habit entirely. In a way many of us are like Pavlov's dogs, conditioned to snack when we sit in our established chair or couch and the TV goes on. To break the habit, read a book or a magazine. Don't turn the TV on at all.

Perhaps play some music. You'll need both hands to hold that book or magazine. Since you're not in the habit of snacking while reading, you probably won't.

I have a personal house rule that calls for zero food or drink in the bedroom. Knowing that I'll snack, sometimes to excess, when I'm under stress and watching TV, I'll head upstairs to the bedroom instead. There I'll either do some reading or TV viewing, but I'm conditioned not to eat in that room. Think about your own snacking and conditioning, and deliberately work to reverse those behavioral patterns.

The American Dim Sum Diet

Dim sum is a wonderful and interesting way to enjoy Chinese food. Essentially, dim sum is a variety of different foods served in small quantities on little plates. The server comes along with a cart, offering this food or that. You either choose to have it or pass. As you eat the foods, which come on different-colored dishes that reflect the prices, plates pile up on the table and at the end of the meal the price is determined by adding up the number of plates.

What I suggest for what I call the "American dim sum diet" has nothing to do with Chinese food, other than the concept of having little servings of this and that. And there's even some solid science behind the idea.

The weight-loss clinic at the University of California Los Angeles (UCLA) medical school uses a similar approach. Its clinicians have developed meal replacements that come in individual servings and a variety of flavors to be mixed with water or diet soda. Each of those packets provides exactly 100 calories and a balance of protein, fat, and carbohydrate. Dieters are instructed to eat eight to nine meal replacements throughout the day. The very low calorie intake, of course, facilitates rapid and satisfying weight loss. By having a mini-meal about every two hours, dieters report much to their amazement that they are never hungry. You can get an inexpensive, virtually identical version of the UCLA 100-calorie meal replacement. Simply do an Internet search for R-Kane Products, Inc. You'll find the packets in a wide variety of flavors.

In my version, I combine the best of UCLA thinking with the unusual Chinese approach to dining out. Instead of meal replacements, my dim sum diet calls for a wide variety of foods eaten throughout the day that have about 100 calories each. Eat eight to nine times a day. You can combine two 100-calorie selections if you wish, but do so no more than twice daily. In addition to those foods, you can also have all the salad greens you can eat dressed with a squeeze of lemon or lime, a splash of flavored vinegar such as balsamic, or a tablespoon of low-cal dressing. Since your food intake will be quite limited, supplement your meals with a multivitamin/mineral tablet. Here's a list of some foods that you might consider.

American Dim Sum Diet Foods	Serving Size	Calories
Seafood		
Salmon	2 oz.	125
Halibut	4 oz.	84
Cooked shrimps	2.5 oz.	100
Scallops	4 oz.	92
Tuna	2 oz.	96
Poultry		
Chicken breast	4 oz.	100
Turkey patty	3 oz.	100
Egg salad	4 oz.	100
Beef		
Extra-lean beef patty	2 oz.	100
Roast beef	3 oz.	111
95% fat-free hot dog	1	54
Pork		
Canadian bacon	2 slices	89
Broiled pork chop	3.5 oz.	150
Lean ham	3.5 oz.	100
Egg (boiled)	1 large	78
Dairy		
Skim milk	8 oz.	86
Plain yogurt	6 oz.	170
Cottage cheese	½ cup	80
Cheddar cheese (low-fat)	1 oz.	55
Vegetables		
Tomato	2.5 oz.	27
Carrots	1 medium	31
Broccoli (raw)	½ cup	12
Cauliflower (raw)	½ cup	13
Bell peppers	½ cup, chopped	14

American Dim Sum Diet Foods	Serving Size	Calories
Fruit		
Apple	1 medium	138
Banana	1 medium	114
Grapefruit	½ medium	118
Kiwifruit	1 medium	76
Peach	1 medium	37
Mango	½ medium	103
Pear	1 medium	98
Nuts		
Dry-roasted almonds	.5 oz.	83
Cashews	.5 oz.	82
Peanuts	.5 oz.	83
Walnuts	.5 oz.	86

Spend a little time in the supermarket and read the labels of other potential foods for the dim sum diet. Check out the calories and serving sizes of soups, canned stews and chili con carne, sardines, canned fish such as salmon and tuna that you can eat right out of the can, breads and cereals, and other foods that you'd enjoy. The wider variety of foods you eat during the weight-loss period, the better, so that you don't become bored.

This diet is especially convenient for people who live alone or those who have unusual eating schedules. An added benefit is the time saved by not having to prepare meals.

As with any diet, it's best to avoid alcoholic beverages for two reasons. First, they obviously are a source of empty calories. Second, they relax inhibitions and might lead you to eat more than you really want to. That said, when my wife went on the diet to lose a few pounds before we headed off on holiday, she replaced one of the mini-meals with a glass of wine in the evening. A 5-ounce serving has about 100 calories. If you'd prefer a cocktail in the evening, an ounce and a half shot of distilled spirits of your choice—gin, vodka, rum—has 90 calories. Mix it with diet soda or water.

This is a rather unusual approach to dieting, I think you'll agree. UCLA has had tremendous success, whether a person wants to lose 10 pounds or 100. To lose very large amounts of weight, obese individuals have followed the program for up to a full year.

Does my dim sum diet fall into the category of "gimmick" diets, as I categorized the previous diets? You bet. On the other hand, there's a lot of UCLA research behind its development. It's a different approach that some people will find helpful.

Learning Portion Control

Virtually every country in the world has developed a guide to healthy eating. Most of them call for eating a wide variety of foods daily to ensure that you get all the nutrients you need.

The foundation of a healthy diet should be a minimum of five servings of fruits and vegetables daily. Personally, I think, and many if not most authorities agree, that the minimum should be up to nine servings a day. You might think that's a huge amount, but two things come into play. First, those plant foods pack very few calories per serving. A serving is a lot less than the average person might guess.

A serving of fruit, as defined by nutritionists, might be one medium apple, banana, pear, or peach. Or it could be two figs, fifteen grapes, two-thirds cup of berries, or a half cup of applesauce. If you're eating dried fruit, a serving would be only two tablespoons of raisins, two medium plums (prunes), or four apple rings. Just 6 ounces of juice constitutes a fruit serving. Starting the day with a glass of juice and some cold cereal with a sliced banana and two-thirds of a cup of berries gives you three servings right off the bat. Grab some raisins or prunes for a snack and you're up to four. Then maybe have sliced mango for dessert at dinner to total five fruit servings for the day.

What about vegetables? Similarly small amounts constitute a serving size. For raw veggies it's one cup. A half cup (4 ounces/ 120 ml) of tomato or other vegetable juices is a serving. A serving of any cooked vegetables would be just one-half cup (4 ounces).

A bowl of soup typically will contain two vegetable servings. What you probably would think to be one serving when you'd see vegetables on a plate would likely be two or, in restaurants, perhaps even three.

The one thing that has shown up in medical studies time and time again, with no contradictory evidence, is that people whose diets are rich in fruits and vegetables are protected against cardiovascular disease, have lower blood pressure, and suffer fewer heart attacks and strokes.

The same holds for whole-grain breads and cereals. Most food guides call for three to four daily servings. In terms of weight control, limit the amount of foods in this category made with refined flour, including pasta, white bread, cakes, and dessert items. Bear in mind that a serving of cooked spaghetti is one cup, which has about 200 calories—not the huge three-cup piles one often sees.

Start thinking the same way about meats and dairy. A serving of meat of any kind is 3½ ounces, about the size of a pack of playing cards or a man's palm. A 1-pound steak is *not* one serving! A serving of cheese of any variety is 1 ounce. Picture a 1-inch-square chunk of cheddar, fontina, or swiss.

Simply learning to judge serving sizes and eating accordingly will help you to lose weight and to maintain that weight loss. Remember that it's a matter of a lifelong change of habits, not just achieving weight loss that rebounds within a few months.

The Essential Weight Control Ingredient

This will be the shortest section in this chapter. Simply stated, weight loss and subsequent weight maintenance *require* physical activity. It's not an option. It is absolutely essential. Every study I've ever read that investigates long-term weight control concludes that regular, fairly strenuous physical activity must go hand in hand with limiting calories.

In our modern society, we have become rather like livestock being readied in a feedlot for the market, with limited movement and unlimited feed. The process by which a previously fit individual becomes overweight and possibly obese is gradual and quite insidious. As one becomes sedentary, muscle is slowly replaced by fat. At first, a person thinks all's well when he or she looks down at the bathroom scales. But, like a well-marbled slab of beef, that person becomes fatter and less muscular.

The only tissue in your body that's capable of burning calories is muscle. Neither skin nor bone nor fat burns energy. Muscle tissue is the furnace of your body. As the percentage of muscle decreases, the ability to expend energy decreases as well. One day, the sedentary individual who has not changed dietary habits by a single calorie since the time he or she was physically fit begins to gain weight. "But doctor," such patients complain, "I'm not eating any more food than I ever have." That's true. But there isn't enough muscle left to burn those same calories, and weight goes up and up and up.

Enough said. It's time to add a regimen of physical activity to your lifestyle. It's so important that I've written an entire chapter on the subject.

Go Ahead, Step on Your Bathroom Scale

Diet experts have argued about this one for years, as long as I've been writing about health and medical matters. Whoops, make that decades instead of years! Some have advised people trying to lose weight to weigh themselves only once a week. Others recommended weighing in every three or four days. Their reasoning was twofold. First, weight loss is a rather slow process and men and women could become discouraged. Second, weight varies slightly from hour to hour and day to day. Thus seeing a 1-pound gain could scuttle a diet.

But two separate recent studies have determined that daily weighing is the "weigh" to go for both weight loss and maintenance. In the first study, done at the University of Minnesota, researchers followed 3,000 overweight or obese men and women for two to three years. Half were in a weight-loss program while the other half were in a program to prevent weight gain. Individuals in the weight-loss program who weighed themselves daily lost twice the weight as did those who weighed in only weekly. The difference was impressive: 12 versus 6 pounds, respectively. People who never weighed themselves *gained* about 4 pounds on average over the course of two years. Conversely, subjects in the weight gain–prevention program who weighed themselves daily *lost* weight.

Researchers in the second study at the Weight Control Center at Brown University in Rhode Island tracked 291 men and women on a weight-maintenance program for seventeen months following an average weight loss of 10 percent of body weight. Of the subjects who did daily weigh-ins, 39 percent gained back at least 5 pounds. That was as good or better than subjects participating in support groups. It was vastly superior to people who weighed themselves less often than daily; 68 percent of them regained at least 5 pounds.

It's really very simple and logical when you think about it. Step on the scale at about the same time of day every day. If you see a slight weight gain, even if that might be from normal daily fluctuation, cut back on the day's food intake. By the next day you'll likely see that unwanted pound gone. That, in turn, encourages you to remain diligent in weight control efforts.

Make the small investment needed to purchase a good-quality scale. Weigh yourself each and every day as part of your weight control and blood pressure control program.

There are many benefits to weight loss beyond good health and blood pressure control, as vitally important as those are. You'll relish hearing friends, relatives, and coworkers tell you how much better you look. Buying new clothes becomes something to look forward to. You'll sleep better, have more energy, experience fewer midafternoon slumps, and simply enjoy life a lot more.

6

Enjoy a Pressure-Friendly Active Lifestyle

There's a single element found in successful weight loss, cholesterol control, stress management, diabetes prevention, and blood pressure maintenance. It's something virtually everyone all over the world who has enjoyed a long life has in common, the factor that all medical authorities agree is essential for both quality and quantity of life. What is this snake oil that appears to be the cure for what ails you? It's physical activity.

Note that I didn't use the term *exercise*. The healthiest men and women in the world aren't necessarily the ones heading off to the gym, but rather those who are physically active most, if not all, days of the week. That's not to say that you should quit your membership to the gym or the health club if you enjoy your workouts on the treadmill or the rowing machine or in classes. My wife, for example, lives a relatively sedentary life as a high school English teacher and in her leisure time plays duplicate bridge. She really doesn't enjoy the outdoors the way I do, but she likes taking exercise classes at the health club. One day she'll do a cycle class, another day it'll be an aerobics class combined with strength and flexibility training. The only sport she loves is snow skiing, which we do together whenever we can.

On the other hand, most of the time I can't wait to get outdoors. I love to hike, ride a bicycle, ski in our local mountains, and, most frequently, walk the up-and-down hills of the golf courses in the canyons where we live. When traveling on business or for pleasure, there's nothing I enjoy more than exploring a new place by walking, often for three, four, or more miles. That said, my work schedule doesn't permit me to do these kinds of recreational activities except on weekends and while on holiday. Most days of the week I condense my activity in the gym, where I walk the treadmill or ride the stationary bike while watching the morning news on a TV monitor.

There are many ways to stay fit and get the physical activity we all need for good health in general and good heart health in particular. Even if you're absolutely set against exercise, whether it's called physical activity or something else, and you define yourself as the ultimate sofa spud, please bear with me through this short chapter. To begin with, I can really relate to you. As a kid in elementary school in the fifties, I flunked the president's physical fitness test while almost everyone else passed. I was always the last one picked for any team sport. No, I am not now nor have I ever been an athlete with a natural attraction to fitness and exercise.

To make matters worse, I went to college in the 1960s, a truly self-destructive era. No one exercised. If anyone was running on campus, you could assume that a cop was chasing him! And after college I became a typical American sedentary office worker.

Looking back on those days, I realize that I was always tired and never felt really well. Yawning every afternoon. Nodding off in meetings, even interesting ones. Not sleeping well at night and having a tough time getting up in the mornings. Lousy at sports— I got into skiing not for the sport but rather for the opportunity to meet girls in the lodge at night. In those days I was actually happy when bad weather kept us off the slopes and in the lodge. I did a lot better with the girls by playing my guitar inside than by skiing, since I was just too weak to carve turns and I skied out of control and fell a lot.

When I had my heart attack and first bypass surgery in 1978 at the tender age of thirty-five, there was no such thing as cardiac rehabilitation and I got no advice about exercise. So if I did anything strenuous, I was scared that I'd have another heart attack.

Then in 1984 my life changed. On July 3, I had my second bypass operation, and three weeks later my cardiologist had me—much against my will—in a rehab program. Little by little I came to life: walking slowly on the treadmill, riding slowly on the bicycle. Everything I did at the beginning I did slowly. But by the end of just six weeks, I felt better than at any time I could recall. By the end of the twelve-week program, I was well on my way to enjoying a life of fitness that I'd never experienced before.

I came to revel in being able to do things that I thought only jocks could do. And on my first ski trip, a year later, I found that much to my surprise, I could actually ski. I was physically able to do the things that I'd learned in lessons earlier. It was fun! It was as if I had a brand-new body.

So, there you are. You're not reading the advice of some Olympic athlete or a wild-eyed fanatic. Simply enough, if I could make the transformation, anyone can!

Looking at things in retrospect, it's too bad that it took a near-catastrophic illness to turn me around. I think of all those years I could have enjoyed more. Sooner would have been better than later, but later was better than never. Now I swear I'll never go back to the old ways. Life is a lot more fun when you have the energy to enjoy it.

Activate Your Healthy Heart

Certainly, this isn't a book for sick people. It's for people who want to prevent problems and for those who want to enjoy their health and their lives. But the one thing that I learned in cardiac rehab that applies to a program of physical fitness for everyone is the word *slowly*. It took years to get to your level of sedentary behavior and lack of fitness, and it'll take time to get going. How long? Ninety days. Give yourself just ninety days. Make a promise, a commitment, to follow the advice in this chapter and I promise, in turn, that by the end of that time you'll be converted for life. You won't want to give up the way you'll feel.

Whether you're trying to prevent a heart attack or a stroke or you want to avoid a second one, exercise just has to be an integral part of the program. Yet the word *exercise* is enough to turn off most people. I can say that because the vast majority of men and women in the United States, Canada, the United Kingdom, Australia and New Zealand, and the rest of the Western world are almost totally sedentary. Thanks to the remote control, they don't even have to walk to the TV to change channels. If you're one of them, you'll be pleased to know that you don't need to exercise in the "no pain, no gain" or "go for the burn" sense of the term. You just need to get active, to just move your body.

Researchers at the Aerobics Institute in Dallas, Texas, wanted to know just how fit people had to be to prevent degenerative diseases, including heart disease. Dr. Steven Blair and his associates studied thousands of men and women, putting them into one of five categories of fitness and regular activity. He expected to see a linear increase in health, a bigger payoff, with every increment of exercise. The results were amazing.

To no one's surprise, people in the top category of fitness were the healthiest. But people in the second-from-the-bottom level, just above the truly sedentary couch potatoes who did absolutely nothing, got almost as much benefit from a minimum of activity as did people in the top tier. The lesson learned: it doesn't take much effort to adequately protect your health.

But how can you measure the activity you need to achieve health and vitality and to prevent heart disease, stroke, and other diseases, including hypertension?

In the past, people were forever talking about heart rates and measuring their pulses. That's really not very practical. Who wants to become obsessed with measuring heartbeats while walking down the block or riding a bicycle on a weekend or, even more to the point, when dancing to a fast beat? As it turns out, this isn't at all necessary. The trick to engaging in effective physical activity comes down to a concept known for many years by exercise physiologists but seldom shared with the rest of the world. It's a way of thinking about activity known as METs, and it's really simple.

When you're completely relaxed, quietly sitting in a chair or lying in bed or on a couch watching television, you're burning just enough energy to keep your internal organs operating and your body alive. That amount of energy, regardless of your age, sex, height, or weight, is one metabolic unit of activity, 1 MET. It's the lowest metabolic level of activity. Get up from that chair to open the window or find a snack, and you've stoked up your body's furnace to 2 METs.

The thinking behind the MET is very logical and easy to understand. When we engage in any physical activity, the heart beats to match demand, to pump out the amount of oxygen-carrying blood needed. Some activities require 50 percent of an individual's maximal capacity. Others call for 60 percent. Still others may need even more. You can determine your own maximal capacity very easily. Simply subtract your age from the number 220. The result is the maximum heartbeats per minute you can achieve without harm. Obviously, we never reach that maximum output.

Let's say you're forty years old. Subtracting 40 from 220 leaves 180. That's your maximal capacity. A normal heart rate, on average, is about 70. So you'd have a long way to go to reach your maximal capacity. Walking briskly might bring your heart rate up to 100 beats per minute. That would be 55 percent of your maximal capacity.

At the same time, our lungs pump oxygen-rich air in and carbon dioxide–laden air out. Again, we have maximal capacities for vigorous breathing. The scientific term for this is VO_2max, referring to the maximum volume of oxygen we can accommodate. That's all you need to know.

Put the two, heart rate and breathing rate, together, and you have a measure of physical performance or level of activity. This measure is termed the *metabolic equivalent*, or MET. The activities of almost every human being can be broken down to the effort required, measured in METs. Take a look at the table on pages 87–89 for a listing of daily activities and their MET ratings.

Remember, I said that *activity*, not *exercise*, is the key to health and fitness. Virtually all medical authorities today agree that walking briskly for thirty to forty minutes a day, at between three and four miles per hour, is sufficient daily exercise. That means about two miles a day, fourteen miles a week. Do just that little bit, or its equivalent, daily, and your heart will thank you for it. That walk will burn from 4 to 6 METs. You can get the same benefit by performing activities requiring half the METs for twice the time or those requiring twice the METs for half the time.

Maybe it's a very busy day, and you just don't have time to take that thirty- to forty-minute walk. Studies have shown that we can break it down to ten- to fifteen-minute chunks of time. The benefit accumulates throughout the day. Or you might concentrate on activities that require the same METs: climbing the stairs instead of using the elevator; picking up the pace of your housework; stepping lively when you need to get from one place to another, whether from your car to an office through the parking lot, down the hallway from one office to another, or doing your grocery shopping and getting the dry cleaning.

Vacuuming the rugs and sweeping the floors can be pretty boring. Here's a tip to make those chores less onerous and good for your heart at the same time. Put on some fast-paced music. Maybe swing, polka, or hip-hop. Whatever you like that gets your toes tapping. Now instead of dancing to that music, do your chores to the beat. Suddenly, you're exercising! You're activating your healthy heart!

Yes, I said that measuring your heart rate isn't necessary, but just to prove a point, put your finger on the side of your neck while you are doing some of those relatively low-MET activities. You'll find that your heart is beating faster and you're breathing more deeply than when you're at rest.

Conversely, you can get the benefit of a low-MET activity by doing activities requiring twice the METs for half the time. Instead of walking at four miles per hour for forty minutes, you can jog at five to six miles an hour for twenty minutes. It's your choice. Hate to jog but love to dance? Get into the habit of square dancing, folk dancing, or swing dancing on a regular basis.

Did you learn to jump rope when you were a kid? That's one of the best forms of cardio exercise. Sound sort of sissy? Think of those boxers training in the gym; every single boxer jumps rope. Do you want to call them sissies to their faces? I think not. Forget those infomercials advertising expensive, inconvenient equipment. You can easily carry a jump rope wherever you go. Take one with you during travel for business or pleasure. Keep one in the office for when you have just five minutes to get in some physical activity. For the best results, buy a good-quality jump rope suited to your height at a sporting goods store.

Most people think that medicine has to taste bad to be effective. They apply that same thinking to activities, concentrating on what might be distasteful to them, what they would call "exercise." Instead, concentrate on the things that are fun for you, whether that might be riding a horse, pedaling a bicycle, rowing a boat or paddling a canoe, or gardening.

The Benefits of Exercise

I could cite chapter and verse from the scientific literature to try to make a convincing argument for the health benefits of exercise. Just lifting the many volumes of books and journals would be a lot of exercise in itself. I'll spare you the details, but here are some of the benefits of regular physical activity.

- You'll feel better. Whatever activity you choose, when the heart and the breathing rates increase to a point that you're breathing deeply and have at least a little perspiration, your body produces a soothing substance called beta-endorphin that's chemically related to morphine. Its calming effect can last the entire day.

   Most psychologists recognize physical activity as one of the best ways to reduce stress. Especially when done on a regular basis, exercise can and will enable you to cope with stress more effectively.

- You'll sleep better. Exercise promotes the release of another chemical, a neurotransmitter known as serotonin. In fact, pharmaceutical companies keep trying to develop drugs that increase serotonin levels to sell as tranquilizers. Exercise is a natural way to produce serotonin to ensure better sleep at night.

- You'll be more productive at work. Most people feel sleepy by midafternoon. Those who regularly exercise find that midday letdowns are a thing of the past. Their stamina increases along with their ability to concentrate. In a survey of highly successful men and women in a number of professions, Dr. Kenneth Pelletier of Stanford University found that virtually all had a regular schedule of physical activity and that they credited their productivity to their exercise habits.

- You'll enjoy sports and leisure recreation more. Whether you play golf, tennis, or any other sport, you'll find that you do it better and enjoy it more when you get regular exercise rather than being a "weekend warrior." That'll probably result in your playing those sports more often, getting even more exercise, and improving your game even more.

- You'll live longer. Here's a little detail that most people find at least moderately interesting. Study after study has shown that physical fitness prolongs life. The more strenuous the activity, the longer one is likely to live.

- You'll control your weight more easily and be able to eat more. Not only do you burn calories during physical activity, but the body's metabolism also remains revved up for hours afterward. In addition, as fitness levels increase, you'll build more lean muscle tissue. Since only muscle tissue can burn calories, acting as the body's furnace, you'll be able to consume more food without gaining weight. You'll find more about this in the weight loss chapter.

- You'll stabilize blood sugar levels and control diabetes. Along with weight loss, regular physical activity can virtually eliminate the symptoms and the health hazards of type 2, non–insulin dependent diabetes. Exercise has an insulinlike effect.

- You'll be less likely to form blood clots that can precipitate heart attacks and strokes. In sedentary people, sudden bursts of activity can cause blood clotting. That may explain why some people have heart attacks when doing unusual activities such as snow shoveling or playing a strenuous game on a weekend. But active men and women are protected against this tendency of blood platelets to form clots. Again, the more you exercise, the greater the protection.

- You'll literally turn back your body's clock. Studies have shown that regular physical activity prevents age-related declines in strength and stamina. For sedentary individuals, six months of endurance exercise reversed thirty years of decline.

Actively Lower Your Blood Pressure

Not only can regular physical activity help to lower blood pressure, but it also takes very little to achieve significant improvements. To determine just how much benefit one can expect, doctors at Tulane University in New Orleans examined the data from fifty-four studies involving a total of 2,419 men and women. Aerobic exercise was associated with what those researchers called "impressive" reductions of nearly 4 points in systolic blood pressure and 3 points in diastolic on average. The higher one's blood pressure at the start of an exercise program, the greater the improvements. But everyone benefits, whether blood pressure is high or normal, and regardless of weight or ethnic origin.

In an editorial published in *The Lancet*, New Zealand physicians summarized what we know about activity levels and blood pressure. Here are the highlights of their summary.

- There were improvements in resting heart rate, total cholesterol, LDL cholesterol, and both systolic and diastolic blood pressure after just six weeks, as stated in a 2005 report.

- One session of exercise at just 40 percent of maximal capacity, the equivalent of moderate walking, can lower blood pressure significantly for up to twenty-four hours.

- After three consecutive periods of activity—let's say, three days of moderate walking—blood pressure is reduced for days, returning to pre-exercise levels only after a week or two of no exercise.

- Blood pressure falls more in hypertensive individuals than in people with normal blood pressure or prehypertension. People with hypertension can achieve systolic blood pressure lowering of 11 points and diastolic blood pressure reductions of 8 points, on average.

- Exercise can slash the ten-year risk of having a heart attack or a stroke by at least 25 percent in the average hypertensive patient, because of the effect on blood pressure and other cardiovascular risk factors.

- Exercising just three times a week, between thirty and sixty minutes a day, is as effective for lowering blood pressure as is exercising five times weekly.

- Breaking down your physical activities into ten-minute segments is effective. You need not exercise continuously for thirty minutes or more at a time.

- Aerobic exercise (walking, bicycling, etc.) appears to be more effective at lowering blood pressure than resistance exercise (weight lifting).

- A study at Indiana University showed that four ten-minute walks daily lowered systolic blood pressure by 6.6 points in pre-hypertensive patients and by 12.9 points in hypertensive people. Breaking up physical activity was actually more effective than a single continuous session. The report was published in the September 2006 issue of *Journal of Hypertension*.

- Increased physical activity, especially vigorous activity that really gets the heart beating faster, lowers the resting heartbeat rate. A heart rate above 80 beats per minute at rest has been linked with an increased risk of heart disease in men and women with hypertension. And a study at the Medical University of South Carolina reported in the *American Journal of Hypertension* in August 2006 showed that the risk of coronary heart disease increased by 50 percent in prehypertensive individuals with resting heart rates more than 80 beats per minute. Increased physical activity can eliminate that risk.

- Low-to-moderate intensities of exercise are as effective, if not more effective, at lowering blood pressure than vigorous exercise is.

So, how does physical activity result in such outstanding pay-offs? It improves blood flow to the heart, arterial flexibility, and arterial function. It slows the development of atherosclerosis and reduces the risk of having heart attacks and strokes.

Take Baby Steps

The ancient Chinese proverb that a journey of one thousand miles begins with a single step has special meaning for people who want to get their blood pressure down. In fact, the worst thing an unfit person could do would be to put on a pair of running shoes and go out for a five-mile jog. Start slowly but surely.

If you have been sedentary for many years, and especially if you're overweight, be sure to talk with your doctor before starting any exercise program. Regardless of your current physical condition, he or she will be delighted to have you increase your activity level and will provide personal guidelines for you.

Consider buying an inexpensive pedometer, one of those little devices worn on a belt, to determine the distance covered in the number of steps, miles, or kilometers. Start wearing it right away. I think you'll be surprised at how many steps you take during a normal day's activities, without any effort to do more. Using that number as a benchmark, gradually increase your activity.

But not all pedometers are accurate, especially the inexpensive ones. A report in the *British Journal of Sports Medicine* gives the Yamax Digiwalker SW-200 high marks for accuracy and reliability. I personally use the Digiwalker SW-401, which counts both steps and miles. The best way to test any pedometer is to measure out a mile on your car's odometer and then walk that exact distance. Also pay attention to the time it takes to walk that mile. That will help you determine just how far you've walked when you're wearing a watch but not a pedometer.

Your goal would be to increase the number of steps taken each day to ten thousand. Remember that all steps count, whether you're out for a brisk walk or simply climbing a flight of stairs at home or at work. Wearing that pedometer acts as a reminder and a motivator. Most men and women find it fun to see each day's improvement over the last. The steps you take start to add up pretty quickly, especially when you make a conscious effort. You'll take more steps when you park your car at the most distant spot when you go shopping. Park your car a block away from work, instead of right at the workplace. Then make it two blocks away. Then three, and so on. Take the stairs instead of the elevator as often as possible. Instead of sitting over a cup of tea or coffee during your break, go out for a brisk ten-minute walk.

Make those steps as much fun as possible. Here's one suggestion for golfers who normally ride a cart. After your drive from the tee, let your buddy take the cart while you walk to the ball with a couple of clubs to take your next shot. On par threes, hit the ball and then walk with (hopefully) your putter or, if necessary, the putter and a wedge. Start by doing just a couple of holes and build up your endurance over time. Be sure to wear your pedometer. Eventually, you'll work your way up to walking a full nine holes or maybe even eighteen holes.

How much is enough? Again, to see improvements in blood pressure, you'd need to take a moderate to brisk walk for thirty minutes or so only three times a week. To achieve weight loss or to maintain your weight, increase that to five or six days weekly. To gain the most benefit for your health in general and your heart in particular, your goal would be to walk about fourteen miles a week or the equivalent in another physical activity.

Remember to make yourself this promise: to stick with a program of increased physical activity for just ninety days. If you do that, you'll feel and sleep better, and you'll never want to quit!

Energy Requirements of Common Activities in METs

1 MET (metabolic equivalent) equals the amount of energy needed when the body is at rest.

Sleeping	Sitting quietly in a chair
Lying in bed	

2 METs equal twice the amount of energy used when at rest.

Standing
Talking
Walking (1 mph)
Reading
Writing

Playing cards
Light housekeeping (dusting)
Typing or word processing
Shaving
Dressing or brushing your hair

2–3 METs

Walking (2 mph)
Playing the piano
Playing golf (electric cart)
Bathing or showering
Washing your hair

Moderate housekeeping (light laundry)
Meal preparation
Bicycling (5 mph)
Bowling

3–4 METs

Walking (3 mph)
Bicycling (8 mph)
Driving a car in light traffic
Climbing stairs slowly

Heavier housework (scrubbing dishes)
Ballroom dancing (foxtrot)
Factory labor

4–5 METs

Walking (4 mph)
Bicycling (8 mph)
Gardening or raking
Light carpentry
Mowing the lawn (power)

Playing badminton or light tennis
Heavy housekeeping (mopping, vacuuming)
House painting
Driving a car in heavy traffic
Washing windows

5–6 METs

Walking (4.5 mph)
Bicycling (10 mph)
Roller-skating
Light shoveling, digging

Golfing (carrying or pulling clubs)
Very heavy housework (scrubbing floors)
Carrying wood or groceries
Social dancing (tango)

6–7 METs

Walking (5 mph)	Mowing the lawn (push mower)
Bicycling (11 mph)	Square dancing, swing dancing
Playing tennis (singles)	Splitting wood
Waterskiing	Snow shoveling
Swimming leisurely	Moving furniture

7–8 METs

Jogging (5 mph)	Playing football
Bicycling (12 mph)	Horseback riding at a gallop
Downhill skiing	Climbing hills (moderate)
Canoeing	Climbing stairs (continuous)
Swimming laps (slow)	Playing tennis (competitive singles)

8–9 METs

Jogging (5.5 mph)	Cross-country skiing
Bicycling (13 mph)	Playing basketball
Swimming laps (fast)	Carrying groceries upstairs

10+ METs

Handball, racquetball, squash, jogging (6 mph and faster)	Climbing hills with a load

7

Reduce Your Stress

Not too many years ago, Western doctors dismissed the idea that mental health and physical health are inextricably linked. They were particularly condescending toward women, who learned to keep their feelings to themselves. The word *hysteria* comes from the Greek word for "woman," and has the connotation of acting emotionally, irrationally, "like a woman." But the reality is that both men and women are indeed affected by their emotions, both positively and negatively.

British researchers have reported in the August 2006 issue of *Heart* that both physical exertion and anger may trigger the onset of chest pain and other cardiac symptoms in patients with heart disease. In fact, emotional states can even precipitate a heart attack.

Many times, I've seen how stress can have a horrible impact on cardiovascular health, and I'm sure you have as well. Have you ever said, "This job is killing me," "That wife/husband of mine is going to give me a heart attack," or "Rush hour traffic makes my blood pressure skyrocket"? Of course, you have. We all have, so you have lots of company.

In the coming pages, I'd like to share some very personal observations, some solid scientific proof of the link connecting emotional states, blood pressure, and heart attacks and strokes, and some suggestions that, yes, you can play a part in controlling some of the stress in your life.

Why hasn't the medical community paid more attention to the

mind/body connection? Part of it comes down to the lack of training in medical schools. And I think one major reason that negative emotional states aren't listed along with more traditional risk factors, such as elevated cholesterol levels, overweight, and high blood pressure, is the inability to directly measure stress, depression, anger, hostility, and anxiety and to quantify those feelings in nice, discrete numbers on the patient's chart.

Fortunately, things seem to be changing. More and more doctors are starting to ask patients about their stress levels, especially when taking medical histories. And they're less likely today to declare either directly or inferentially that "It's all in your mind" when counseling men and women. Medical schools are teaching about the mind/body connection. Typically, they've come up with a new word to legitimize the emerging new field: *psychoneuro-immunology.* This big term simply states that there is a link between the mind, the nervous system, and the many ways the body works.

Let me start with a few personal observations. I mentioned earlier that my father had severe hypertension and that he died of a heart attack. Or it might have been a stroke, since no autopsy was ever performed. One way or the other, there's no doubt in my mind that Dad's fatal cardiovascular event that terrible day in December 1969 was precipitated by overwhelming stress.

My father had been one of those lucky guys who really loved his work as a neighborhood pharmacist. He was dearly beloved by his customers and he loved them back. Although he put in long hours in the store, he never really thought about it as "work" in a negative way—until a robbery at the pharmacy resulted in the savage stabbing of his assistant pharmacist, a man who had been like a brother to him for many, many years. Although Vince survived the attack, my Dad's feelings about the store changed dramatically. Every time he opened the door in the morning, he was filled with dread at having to be at the scene of the crime.

In a matter of months, his health deteriorated and he visibly aged. My mother, brother, and I, along with others, tried to convince Dad to simply get out of that store, fearing it would literally kill him. And it did. Whether it was a heart attack or a stroke doesn't matter. Dad had underlying cardiovascular disease and hypertension and the stress was the precipitating factor that led to his death. I still miss him horribly.

In my own case, in 1978, I suffered from overwhelming stress caused by a personal problem that I found impossible to resolve. I couldn't get it out of my mind. In retrospect, I think my blood pressure was probably skyrocketing. And there were factors that had led to my underlying heart disease, including too many years of smoking two packs of cigarettes a day, living a mostly sedentary existence, and eating a diet high in saturated fat and cholesterol. I was also unable to talk with anyone about my problems. I kept my fears and anxiety bottled up and the pressure built up to that day in May nearly three decades ago when I had my heart attack. I was lucky. Unlike my dad, I survived.

Next there's my own brother. Tom has always been a happy-go-lucky guy who liked his work and was so good at it that he didn't have to spend much time working to earn his very nice salary. Then his luck ran out. Financial woes became overwhelming and were always on his mind. It wasn't much of a surprise when he called from the hospital telling me that he had had a heart attack.

I've read case histories in the medical literature detailing how business executives in the cardiac care unit of the hospital, where they were recovering from heart attacks, confided that in a perverse way they were happy. Why? Because being in the hospital with no access to a telephone and with no visitors other than immediate family meant the first "vacation" they'd had in years and the first time they were relieved of the responsibilities that had led to a malignant level of stress.

And then there was a friend of mine, a mathematics teacher in middle school working with kids eleven to thirteen years old. On the golf course on weekends, he'd tell me that while he loved his work and loved the contributions he knew he was making toward having a lasting impact on those boys and girls, he found the pressures and the time constraints to be onerous. Fast forward: Chris suffered what turned out to be three, not one but three, simultaneous strokes. Happily, he survived, but the ill effects of that event forced him to take early retirement owing to disability.

I'm not trying to scare you. That's not my style. Rather, I'm trying to impress upon you just how important a role your emotional health plays on your cardiovascular health. If anything I've said thus far has made an impression, has reminded you of yourself, then you're now ready to learn just how the mind/body connection can lead to hypertension and what you can do to stop or at least slow down the insidious process.

It's rather ironic that our language is replete with terms and phrases such as *heartache*, *heartbreak*, *heartfelt remark*, *heartless behavior*, *be still, my beating heart*, and so forth. We intuitively know that the heart is more than a chunk of muscle that pumps blood.

The World Health Organization (WHO) Global Burden of Disease Survey estimates that by 2020, major depression will be second only to ischemic heart disease in the degree of disability it will bring to people suffering from severely negative emotions. We're polluting our planet's earth, air, and water. And we're polluting our bodies with stress, anxiety, anger, hostility, and depression.

Job Stress and Blood Pressure

It'll come as no surprise to anyone who dislikes his or her job or feels a lot of stress at work that the greatest number of heart attacks occur on Mondays. Stress, it turns out, is indeed a killer. That's especially true when one's job demands high performance but offers little in the way of control. The Japanese have a chilling term for this: *karoshi*. It means "death from overwork."

Investigators at the University College London evaluated data from more than ten thousand civil service workers. Compared with subjects who didn't report job-related stress, people who told of work stress three or more times over the span of the fourteen-year study had double the risk of metabolic syndrome, which includes elevated blood pressure along with other heart-related risk factors. People complaining of work stress typically were in jobs with high demands and low levels of control.

Canadian researchers studied 8,395 white-collar workers in

Quebec City from 1991 to 1993 and followed up with 84 percent of the participants seven and a half years later to assess the impact of job strain. Compared with a similar group of workers not exposed to the same levels of work-related stress, the subjects who were under continuous job strain had an increase in systolic blood pressure equivalent to that expected from aging and sedentary behavior. Put in other words, the job stress those workers experienced was equal in its ill effects to aging seven and a half years or being sedentary for that period of time.

To better understand who is at risk, let's consider the lucky people who are not. Orchestra conductors tend to live long lives and continue their careers well after most folks would want to retire. Why? They love their work, they are truly passionate about their art, and despite potential frustration when the violinist or the cello player doesn't hit a note just right, they have enormous control over their situations. Conductors are absolute bosses. Some people might even call them tyrants.

On a lighter note, consider entertainers such as Bob Hope and many others who live well into their nineties. They, too, seldom retire. They enjoy their work and that work gives meaning to their lives. And why not? No one tells them what to do or when to do it. Sure, such men and women put high demands on themselves, but they are in control of their lives and their careers.

In the business world, the same can be said for top management. The highest-level executives make decisions and tell others to carry them out. Ultimately the real work falls on the shoulders of a low-echelon person who carries a large burden, never seems to catch up with the day's work, and has no control over how that work is to be done. He or she goes home each night thinking about the work still on the desk and knowing that tomorrow there will be even more.

Now let's intensify that scenario. The trip home from work is far from an idyllic ride through a beautiful valley filled with flowering shrubs and birds in the sky. No, it's bumper-to-bumper traffic with white knuckles on the steering wheel. After thirty, forty, or more minutes of near collisions and road rage, our worker finally comes home.

Forget the tableaus of 1950s-style television. Instead, there are crying children, appliances that have broken down, bills in the mail, and a spouse whose day has been just as trying.

Doctors don't really understand why, but women tend to endure such stressful lifestyles more successfully than men do. It's the men whose blood pressures go up and up. But, sadly, that's changing. Now that women are trying to balance careers with the demands of raising children and managing the household, often with little or no help from their husbands, they, too, are becoming hypertensive. Surely, that's not what the early feminists seeking equality had in mind.

Want to know the worst possible scenario? Combine job strain with poor marital relationships, and you have the formula for blood pressures going through the roof. That was the conclusion of researchers at the University of Toronto in Canada. They found that the amount of support received at home in a relationship is critical to a person's health.

Because we live at a time when both men and women must work, or at least both want to work, outside the home, we have to learn how to survive the situation. This means taking a bit of time, ideally away from the children, to actually talk. Ask about your spouse's day. Give your partner the chance to vent his or her frustrations.

Does that sound completely unrealistic? It can be done. It's a matter of recognizing the importance of relying on each other.

Here's my suggestion. At a time when things aren't at their very worst, when both of you are relatively at ease, think about setting a time each day to sit down for as little as ten minutes just to talk. And listen. Come on now, be honest with yourself. You find the time to spend hours and hours each week staring at the TV. Can't you assign ten minutes a day to improve your relationship and at the same time vent the emotions that can lead to hypertension?

Here's the reality. Job strain raises blood pressure during your working hours. At first, the body—notably, your arteries—is quite resilient. When the whistle blows and it's time to quit for the day, blood pressure returns to normal. But when rises in blood pressure occur day after day, week after week, that resiliency diminishes and blood pressure eventually fails to return to normal. Picture your arteries as rubber bands that are repeatedly stretched to their limits. At some point the elasticity is gone and the rubber band breaks.

The Type-A Personality and Beyond

In the 1970s, two doctors in San Francisco, California, revolutionized the field of cardiology and added a term to the vocabulary worldwide. They described people who were angry, time-obsessed, and driven as having the *type-A personality*. These people were said to be at greater risk of developing heart disease and hypertension and of having heart attacks and strokes. But there was always something wrong with that picture.

If everyone who is driven by his or her career aspirations and by the need for success has a heart attack or a stroke, how can we have successful businessmen, doctors, entertainers, and world leaders? And how is it that the most successful people actually live quite long lives? And if some people weren't obsessed with time and deadlines, newspapers could never hit the stands—and this book would never have been written!

It turns out that the concept of the type-A personality had it only half right. What can be fatal is the anger and the hostility that may develop out of stressful situations, especially in people prone to such negative emotions. A long-term study of more than a thousand men found that those who had angry or irritable responses to stressful situations were three times more likely to be diagnosed with heart disease and five times more likely to suffer a heart attack before the age of fifty-five. Another investigation showed that women with heart disease who were hostile had double the risk of having a heart attack or dying from heart problems than did women who weren't hostile.

Most of the time, the process is slow and insidious. Hypertension and the resultant heart attacks and strokes don't develop overnight. But in our stress-ridden society, anger and hostility can kill suddenly and dramatically. It was a California psychologist who coined the term *road rage* to describe the behavior displayed when too many cars clog that state's roads and freeways. It sounds absurd, but this scenario has been played out too many times: one driver is cut off by another guy, he flashes an obscene gesture in anger, and the other driver pulls out a gun and shoots. Hey, it's not just men. I've seen women screaming at each other over a contested parking place in a shopping mall.

Exaggerated instances? Such behaviors occur every day. Going back to the worker with huge job demands and little control, we now have the term *going postal* to describe the sometimes fatal anger and fury that can boil over. That term was coined when post office workers solved their problems with blazing guns.

Every country has its problems. A Japanese study classified workers by the amount of overtime they put in. Investigators found that while there were no significant differences in conventionally measured blood pressure levels, people who worked an average of sixty or more extra hours a month had higher twenty-four-hour blood pressure levels. Both blood pressure and heart rate were higher when workers were accumulating overtime.

In England, a study was conducted with ten thousand civil servants. People in the lowest grades of the administration were at the highest risk for cardiovascular diseases. During work hours, their blood pressure went up. And the lower the person was on the administrative ladder, the higher the pressure went.

As human beings, we're not the only creatures who respond very badly to stress. Hans Selye, a Canadian researcher credited with being the father of the study of stress, used ordinary house mice as his test subjects. As his mouse population grew in a confined space, males fought more aggressively over territory, sometimes to the death. And females ceased to reproduce.

How Emotions Kill

Stress and other negative emotions affect our bodies in very tangible, physiological ways. As one example, especially for people who are prone to irregular heart rhythms, mental stress can trigger dangerous disruptions in the heartbeat. Those disruptions can be enough to cause a heart attack. But even people without existing arrhythmias can be at risk, as has been tragically demonstrated at such disasters as the World Trade Center attack in New York. Following that catastrophe, cardiovascular events such as heart attacks and strokes multiplied.

Mental stress can trigger a lack of blood flow to the heart, thus heightening the risk of death in people who already have clogged arteries. Such mental stress increases oxygen demand because blood pressure and heart rate go up. At the same time, stiffened arteries resist the greater blood flow and coronary arteries in the heart constrict, further decreasing the blood supply.

Mental stress also causes the inner layer of the blood vessels to constrict, which may increase the risk of sudden cardiac death. Sudden stress leads to *endothelial dysfunction*, the medical term for a malfunction of the arterial linings, and the artery's ability to dilate is impaired. Swiss researchers found a significant decrease in blood vessel dilation after mental stress. Diastolic blood pressure shot up from 83 to 96 and heart rate rose from 63 to 81 beats per minute.

Doctors can actually measure the chemicals that rush into your bloodstream when you feel stress, anger, and hostility. Cortisol, adrenaline, noradrenaline, and others not worth your memorizing or even hearing about all raise blood pressure. Early in our evolution, those chemicals prepared us for fight or flight. Cavemen, I'm sure, experienced tremendous anxiety when they encountered vicious animals that were intent on turning them into dinner. But once the fight or flight was over, those early men leaned against a rock or a tree and relaxed. Later they might have bragged about their victory while sitting around the fire. In other words, their stress was not relentless, as ours may be today. That's a curse of modern times for too many men and women.

According to doctors working in Sweden, hypertensive men who don't manage stressful situations well may be at increased risk of having strokes. Those researchers followed 238 hypertensive men from 1982 through 1996. They concluded that men who fail to find successful strategies to manage a situation or solve a conflict are in trouble. Such individuals don't work methodically. They try a number of strategies without giving them enough time to see if they work. In the long run, that kind of behavior creates wear and tear on the body.

Let's look at it in a step-by-step fashion. You find yourself under mental stress at work but don't find a way to cope with that stress. Your blood pressure goes up during those working hours. The stressful situation is repeated daily. At first, your blood pressure returns to normal when the work whistle blows. Eventually, your blood pressure remains elevated even during nonworking hours. Now you're formally hypertensive. As a hypertensive patient, you are now more at risk of having a heart attack or a stroke when faced with a sudden, intense emotion of whatever sort. That risk is, of course, multiplied many times by a concurrent elevation of cholesterol, a sedentary lifestyle, cigarette smoking, diabetes, and other factors. That's not a good crystal ball to gaze into, is it?

Learn to Control Your Stress

You have a tremendous capability of controlling the mind/body connection. It takes no special talent, and you don't have to become a meditating monk living far from the pressures of civilization. Here's one simple demonstration. Close your eyes for just a moment and think about a lemon. Picture yourself slicing that lemon and watching the juices flow. You can smell that lemony aroma. Now imagine picking up a slice and putting it into your mouth and sucking on the tart, juicy fruit.

What happened? Your mouth started to water. Unless you have some sort of underlying disorder that limits your ability to salivate, it's almost impossible not to have your mouth water when you think about that juicy lemon. In a very real way, your thoughts have had a dramatic effect on your body.

The mind is a wonderful, awesome thing. Try not to think of elephants. Really. Put elephants completely out of your mind. When trying not to do so, you just can't seem to make those big creatures go away. And we've all had times when we can't get the words or the melody of a song out of our minds.

Here's an experiment to try when you get a home blood pressure monitor, which I really hope you will do. Put the cuff around your arm and measure your pressure. Note the reading. Now think about something that happened in your life either recently or a while back that really made you angry. Dwell on that negative experience for two or three minutes. Then measure your blood pressure again. Almost certainly the numbers will be higher.

The good news is that you can do just exactly the opposite, whether you're hooked up to a monitor or not. It might sound strange, but thinking happy thoughts at times when a situation would normally generate anger or hostility can medicate your mind. Pleasant thoughts cause the release of relaxing neurotransmitters in the brain. This is not wishful thinking, but rather a scientific fact that has been documented by high-tech instruments taking photos of the brain and showing the very positive effects of such mental manipulations.

So try this experiment for yourself. Sit down with the blood pressure monitor in place, the cuff around your upper arm. Push the button, take your blood pressure reading, and make a note of it. Now close your eyes for two to three minutes, and concentrate on breathing in and out, slowly and deeply. Imagine your chest as an inflating and deflating balloon. After that two- to three-minute breathing exercise, take your blood pressure again. You'll be amazed at the improvement.

Take that two- to three-minute "vacation" a few times daily, especially when you're under stressful conditions, and you'll make a significant improvement in your blood pressure.

As with any other endeavor, learning to cope with stress takes some effort and your capabilities will increase with practice. The coping suggestions that I'll give you in the balance of this chapter can have a very real, physical effect on your brain and your emotional status. And they can help you to control your blood pressure, just as surely as prescription antianxiety medications can. Both medications and the coping suggestions will increase levels of sero-tonin, "the happy neurotransmitter," in the brain.

I've proved this time and time again with friends and relatives who were having attacks of hiccups. Hiccups, you ask? What do hiccups have to do with blood pressure? Well, nothing, really. But what I'm about to describe is a fairly dramatic demonstration of just how well one can control one's bodily functions.

Hiccups are caused by spasms of the diaphragm that are followed by a sudden closing of the glottis, an opening in the back of the throat, causing an interruption of air flow and resulting in the characteristic sound. Hiccups follow an irritation of the nerves that control the respiratory muscles, particularly the diaphragm. Many things, from swallowing hot or irritating foods or beverages to bouts of joyous laughter, can cause them. We've all heard of this cure or that: holding one's breath, putting a paper bag over the head, being startled. Sometimes they work; most times they don't. But trust me, my cure is 100 percent effective each and every time.

It demonstrates how you can indeed affect a malfunctioning part of the body. You can, in this case, stop the spasms of the diaphragm and, poof, the hiccups are gone. So, here we go. Please don't roll your eyes or think this is in the realm of weirdo-hippy gobbledygook. Try this technique the next time you or someone else gets the hiccups.

Find a place where you can be alone. You can't concentrate effectively if you're with a group of people or even just two. Ideally, turn the lights down, not necessarily off. Sit with your back straight up and your legs crossed, with your arms on top of your legs and your palms up and fingers gently bent. Yeah, I know, you're already starting to think Indian guru nonsense. Again, bear with me. Don't knock it until you try it.

Close your eyes. Take in a deep, deep breath and think of your chest as a balloon that's filling to maximum capacity. When you think you've taken in as much air as you can hold, "sip" in a little more. Then hold your breath as long as you can, with your back still upright. Now slowly, slowly release your breath. As you do so, again imagine your body as a balloon that's had a puncture and the air is gradually leaking out, causing the balloon to deflate. As you exhale, allow your body to fall forward, chest toward your legs. At the point when you think all the air is out, puff a couple more breaths out. Then very slowly begin to breathe air back into that balloon, inflating it as your back returns to the upright position. Think about that air. Feel how your body inflates and then deflates. Do that a few times. Feel yourself totally relaxing. You're thinking about nothing but your breathing in and out, in and out. Then, Bingo! Your hiccups will be gone.

This technique has never failed, and everyone I've ever showed it to has become a zealot, teaching others how to do it. Try it the next time you get hiccups.

You'll find that you get an unexpected bonus. You'll wind up feeling remarkably relaxed. That leads me to why I shared this tip with you. You don't have to wait for the hiccups to get that relaxed feeling. You can do this routine every day. And, indeed, you should do so. The more often you try it, the better you'll get at achieving a remarkable state of relaxation.

With a bit of practice, you'll find that just as you're able to stop a bout of hiccups, you can stop an episode of anxiety. But don't wait for an anxious, stressful moment. As with any other skill, this one takes some practice. So do your practicing when you're not anxious, upset, or angry. I like to think of it as taking mini-vacations during the day. No matter where you are—at work, at home, or elsewhere—you can find a quiet place to gain a sense of peace.

If you wait until you're in a bad mood, without first practicing the technique, you'll be too upset to achieve self-soothing. If you've done it a number of times before a situation occurs when you really need it, you'll find that you can breathe your anger away. Really and truly.

Even if you're sitting at a conference table with business associates—or family members, for that matter—you can at least do some deep breathing. Remember that old saw "Count to ten before losing your temper"? Try taking ten deep, deep breaths in and out, thinking about your breathing, to relieve some of your anxiety.

As time goes on, you may very well come to appreciate the soothing feeling you can achieve with that kind of breathing. You might graduate to reserving five or ten minutes once or twice a day simply to take a mini-vacation. What you're doing is a type of meditation. And while you might balk at the very word *meditation*, isn't meditation better than, and preferable to, medication?

You might also want to try what's called "mindfulness." Unlike the kind of meditation that most people are, if not familiar with, at least aware of, mindfulness is a conscious effort to think or to concentrate. In meditation, people try to clear their minds of all thought, and that's not everyone's cup of tea. It's surely not mine. I prefer to be mindful of, say, my breathing. Or, while taking a walk, I'll concentrate and really think about the mechanics of walking: striding forward while balancing on the back leg, then flexing the back foot and pushing that leg forward as the other leg moves to the back, and so forth. Or think about my heart beating in my chest and how it's pumping blood through the miles of arteries to every nook and cranny of my body. Or look into the sky and marvel at the clouds. You can do this even while you're working at home or at some task—unless, of course, you're operating a chain saw or a punch press in a factory!

Psychologists have developed a technique called biofeedback, in which one concentrates on the heartbeat or breathing. The feedback comes from a machine that registers blood pressure, heart rate, or both. The apparatus and the training can be expensive, but some people find biofeedback to be very helpful.

There's a far less expensive tool I can recommend that helps you to become effective with relaxed breathing. It's called RESPeRATE and is a device that runs you through breathing exercises and has been clinically proven to be beneficial in controlling both stress and hypertension. You can learn more about RESPeRATE and can order it online at www.high-blood-pressure-help.com.

Four studies detailing the effectiveness of RESPeRATE were presented at the American Society of Hypertension Annual Scientific Meeting in May 2006. The studies demonstrated RESPeRATE's ability to reduce resistance in narrowed blood vessels, thus facilitating blood flow and lowering blood pressure. A review article on seven clinical studies with RESPeRATE was published in *Medscape General Medicine* in December 2006. Details of those studies as well as an in-depth look at how RESPeRATE works to lower blood pressure can be viewed at www.resperate.com/MD.

What are some other ways of coping with stress? Almost all doctors and psychologists agree that one of the best ways is exercise. If *exercise* is a dirty word to you, think of it merely as physical activity. In other words, you don't have to go to a gym and run endlessly on a treadmill. Relaxing physical activity can be anything you enjoy doing. Studies comparing the mechanics of various activities have shown that one can achieve similar "work" when gardening, dancing, bicycle riding, walking through the woods, opting to walk rather than use a cart on the golf course, or even housecleaning at a rapid pace. My wife has learned that when I get angry about something, I tend to clean up the kitchen or do some other chore at a nearly breakneck pace. Of course, she doesn't mind a bit!

Then there's "work" versus work. One man's work is another man's pleasure—or hobby, as it were. Probably the last thing a professional carpenter would want to do in his spare time is woodworking. But for a number of men I've known who make their living in a court of law, a business office, or a hospital, woodworking in the basement, perhaps making a birdhouse, is an absolute joy. Try putting together a jigsaw puzzle. Or get a pair of binoculars and a bird book to identify the birds in your backyard. Whatever the hobby might be, find something you can enjoy to take your mind off things that cause stress.

By the way, watching TV is not a good way to relax. I won't go into unnecessary technical details, but the brain does not relax when gazing at the screen in the same way it might when solving a crossword puzzle or reading a book or a magazine. Limit the time you spend in front of the tube and expand your activities to other things.

Are you an animal lover? Many studies have confirmed that petting a dog or taking it for a walk makes one's blood pressure plummet. Some doctors and psychologists have gone so far as to strongly recommend that patients get pets. Many care facilities for the elderly have taken in dogs and cats to help residents stay relaxed.

Here's something to really think about. Are you nice to yourself? How well do you treat yourself? Most men and women do far more for others than they do for themselves, and they put themselves at the lowest priority. Do something nice for yourself, not just once in a while but on a regular basis. My wife really likes to get a facial. I prefer a massage, which I schedule on late Friday afternoons every two weeks. It's something I look forward to and is a nice way to end the workweek and start the weekend on a relaxing note. Too expensive? There are massage schools that offer cut-rate services from students. On Sunday mornings, my wife loves to make her bowl of oatmeal and work a crossword puzzle while eating it, no matter how much work she has waiting to do that day. And on those weekends you'll seldom find me in the office; I'll be out hiking, on the golf course, or fishing with some friends. While I'm doing one of those things, my wife will be playing a game of duplicate bridge; she's a life master and takes the game quite seriously. Both my wife and I work very hard, putting in long hours every week, but we make sure there's time for fun and games! We deserve it, and so do you.

Can you find stress relief in a pill? Certainly there are several prescription drugs such as Valium (diazepam) your doctor could suggest. But all come with a variety of potential side effects, the least of which would be drowsiness. You want to relax, not collapse! I'm happy to say that once again there is a completely natural alternative that I've used myself with great satisfaction.

L-theanine is an amino acid found in green tea. Over the years, many men and women have achieved a soothing effect from sipping a cup of green tea, and L-theanine appears to be the active ingredient that reduces stress and facilitates relaxation without drowsiness. This natural substance is absorbed in the small intestine and crosses the blood-brain barrier where it is absorbed into the brain. There it stimulates the production of restful and relaxed alpha brain waves similar to that achieved in meditation. There is a corresponding reduction in beta waves. One remains completely alert but far more relaxed.

You should experience the soothing effects of L-theanine within thirty minutes, and those effects can last anywhere from eight to twelve hours. There are no food or drug interactions, and you can take the amino acid at any time. When you take L-theanine about an hour before bedtime, you may experience a better, more restful night's sleep and be prepared for the coming day and more capable of coping with the day's stresses. To achieve the best effects for taking the edge off a particularly stressful day, take between 100 mg and 200 mg. Note that if you're already feeling calm, you won't notice any difference. But if you're on edge or even feeling a bit jittery after drinking coffee, you see the benefits. There have been literally dozens of clinical studies that document the safety and efficacy of L-theanine as a calming agent. I now use it on a fairly regular basis. For example, I enjoy the lift I get from a cup or two of strong coffee in the morning but not the jitters that L-theanine smoothes out. And when faced with stressful deadlines and other demands of life, I find that the amino acid gives me the calming effect I want without the ill effects of a drug. Of course I still practice other relaxation techniques including deep breathing and physical activity.

L-theanine is sold on the Internet and in various health food stores and pharmacies under a number of brands. Read the labels to see the name Suntheanine to assure a good form of the amino acid produced by the Japanese company Taiyo.

The next time you find yourself steaming with anger over something, ask yourself this simple, five-word question: *Is it worth dying for?* There's no doubt in my mind that if my father knew that the stress he was experiencing in the months before his death would lead to that fatal heart attack or stroke, he would have locked the store and never gone back. He could have eventually sold the pharmacy and made a decent living as a pharmacist working elsewhere.

Is work killing you? Either find a way to cope with that job or get a different job. Does your spouse make you angry far too often? Get counseling. Do certain issues have you losing sleep at night? Perhaps there's a friend or a clergyman you can confide in. Speak with your physician about therapy, prescription drugs, or both. The list could go on and on. Only you know your "triggers." And only you can seek a solution if the coping mechanisms I've suggested just aren't enough and if you know your blood pressure is going up. Take the pressure off your heart.

Keep those five words in mind: *Is it worth dying for?* You know that the answer is, "Hell, no!"

8

Time to Quit Smoking

You've heard all the statistics. Smoking kills more than 19,000 men and women every year. In the United States that number is 400,000 deaths annually, 180,000 of which are due to heart attacks and strokes. A British study calculated that the average smoker burns up $160,000 in a lifetime. Numbers and more numbers. Yada, yada, yada.

Cigarette smoking triples the risk of having a heart attack. But, as noted in the August 19, 2006, issue of *The Lancet*, the risk of having a heart attack increases with *all* forms of tobacco usage, not just cigarettes.

As a former smoker myself, I know just how you feel. And believe me right from the start, I'm not going to pontificate. I'm not going to try to convince you to quit. You've gotten that from your doctor, your husband or wife or boyfriend or girlfriend, your children, your friends. But if you're ready to quit, I'll help you do it. And I'll point to others who can give you more assistance.

The reality is that people who successfully quit really *want* to quit. They haven't been talked into it or frightened into it. They've finally hit the wall and truthfully said to themselves, "I *want* to quit." Just saying "I should quit" won't do it. I hope you now want to quit, just as I really wanted to twenty-six years ago when I finally said good-bye to my friend and lover, my cigarette.

Nonsmokers just don't understand smokers. "Hey, it's just a

habit, get over it!" "Millions of other smokers have quit; so can you." "If you really loved me, you'd quit."

As one smoker said to me during a coffee break at work when we were both puffing away, "I can't imagine living without smoking." I couldn't, either. Smoking was part of my life. Hell, my cigarettes were my best friends, only more dependable—they were there whenever I wanted to celebrate, grieve, or anything in between. More than just a friend, my cigarette was my lover. Paul Simon sang, "There must be fifty ways to leave your lover," but I hadn't found one that worked for me.

Like Mark Twain once famously said, "It's easy to quit, I've done it many times." But until the time I finally quit for good, my quitting never lasted more than a couple of days.

Trained as a journalist in college, I was forever in a cloud of blue smoke, my own and that of others. Coffee and cigarettes were our fuel. We couldn't imagine writing without both, especially the cigarettes. My brand was Marlboros, and when I was a kid about eighteen years old I actually thought about getting the Marlboro Man's tattoo on the back of my hand just like his. It looked so cool when he'd light his weed from a glowing stick he pulled out of the campfire in those 1960s TV ads. Hey, forget the fact that the Marlboro Man died of lung cancer.

Even my major professor in physiology during my graduate training was a smoker. He often smoked while giving his lectures. I learned years later that he had died of a heart attack.

After graduating from college I had a terrific job, making quite a bit of money for a young guy. I couldn't pick up the phone without lighting a cigarette. Or attend a meeting. Or have a cup of coffee. I remember saying that I'd gladly write a check for $1,000 to someone who could give me an injection or a pill so I could wake up in the morning a nonsmoker. Those were the days when $1,000 was big money, by the way. But I also said I wouldn't take a check for $1,000 to quit, since I knew I couldn't.

Did you practice smoking in front of a mirror as a kid when you first started to smoke? I did. I learned to "French inhale" the smoke into my nostrils from my mouth. I tried to look like Europeans in the movies. And I loved playing with my Zippo lighter. I loved it!

The day I came home to my apartment after being discharged from the hospital in 1978 after my first bypass surgery, I made a martini and lit a Marlboro. After all, my surgeon told me I had something wrong, and he fixed it. He said to enjoy my life and forget all about the surgery. Later on my cardiologist, an internationally renowned man, said that the six or so cigarettes I smoked daily (I had coincidentally cut down during that time) probably weren't too bad if they helped me to relax at the end of the day. The medical consensus sure has changed since then!

I quit one day in July of 1979. By that time I not only knew I should quit, I really wanted to quit. I didn't want to smoke those forty cigarettes a day; I had to. They were controlling me, I wasn't controlling them. It was impossible for me to smoke only the cigarettes that I actually enjoyed. Getting deathly ill was my lucky break. I woke up one morning with a horrible sore throat. I tried to inhale my first cigarette of the day and the smoke felt like razor blades. So I thought that I wouldn't smoke for the rest of the day. In fact, I put the last of my pack in the garbage disposal. The next morning, still sick as a dog, I went out and bought another pack. I lit one and it was just as bad. Okay, I said, one more day without smoking. And I threw the pack away and went back up to the apartment and into bed. That went on for almost a week. Then I thought, Hey, this is the longest I've ever gone without a smoke. I wondered whether I could do just "one more day."

Like an alcoholic who's gone to Alcoholics Anonymous, I lived my life going "one more day" without smoking for the next few weeks. Back at work, I mouthed a toothpick or sucked hard candies at meetings at work. And I adopted quite a few tricks and techniques to living life without cigarettes. Was it tough? Probably the most difficult thing I've ever done. Did it work? I've been a non-smoker since that July day in 1979.

In this chapter I'll share some of the things that helped me to succeed. And I'll detail the information I've gained by doing research with major health groups, I'll compare methods of quitting, and I'll examine some of the aids that didn't exist back in '79. If you've finally come to that time in your life when you *want* to quit, when you're literally sick and tired of smoking, and when you finally admit to yourself that you no longer smoke for pleasure, you smoke because you *have* to smoke, and that down deep inside you *hate* those cigarettes as much as or more than you love them, I know I can help.

When *Not* to Quit

In an ideal world, any time would be a good time to quit smoking. But we live in a real world. Don't try to do it when you're under an unusual amount of stress because you're likely to fail, and that'll just convince you that you can't quit. If you were served with divorce papers today, it might not be the best time to quit. The flip side of the coin is when you're on a vacation. You might think that'd be a great time to leave the cigarettes behind, but the harsh facts are that you'd be edgy, irritable, and miserable, and you'd make everyone around you unhappy as well. Don't spoil that vacation.

Instead, pick a day like any other day. A typical day, nothing unusual. Hey, we're all under a certain amount of stress at work and at home, so you can't expect to have a stress-free day that would be the idyllic time to stop smoking. Even if you did, that wouldn't necessarily prepare you for ordinary days.

Many organizations and support groups suggest picking a day on the calendar some time in the future. Some day next week or next month. Start preparing for your "quit date" by stocking up on stuff to keep your mind off the cigarettes and things to play with to keep your hands occupied. Lay in a supply of toothpicks, hard candies, chewing gum, bottled water, worry beads, nicotine patches, and healthy snacks. Tell all your friends and family in advance. The problem with that sort of planning is that you're very likely to postpone that quit date and wind up feeling embarrassed to the point that it'll discourage you from future attempts. But many people have indeed used that planning technique successfully.

A British study indicates that the best approach might be to simply decide one day, That's it, I quit. And just do it. Starting that day. No putting it off anymore. That's sort of like jumping right into the pool of cold water rather than dipping in a toe, then the foot, and so on. In retrospect, that's just what I did. I woke up sick, the cigarette hurt my throat, and I decided to quit. In the past I'd made bets with my college roommates, promised a girlfriend that I'd quit, made plans to do so when school was out, or whatever. For me, at least, that never worked. In talking with fellow quitters, the majority said they made a spontaneous decision one day and never smoked again.

Ultimately, it will be your decision as to when you quit and how. In the meantime, let me point out the effect that your next cigarette will have on your body. Smoking just one cigarette can cause a sudden change in how well your heart beats. Your blood pressure goes up. Your arteries constrict. These are not good things to have happen. But let's look at some of the good things that you'll experience when you do quit.

The Benefits of Quitting Smoking

Just twenty minutes after your last cigarette, your blood pressure starts going down. Your heart rate gets slower. And your hands and feet start to feel warmer, demonstrating the almost immediate improvement in circulation. Within eight hours, carbon monoxide levels in your blood drop to normal, replaced by invigorating oxygen. By the end of the first day, in a mere twenty-four hours, your chances of suffering a heart attack or a stroke go down. After two smoke-free days your nerve endings return to normal function and your ability to smell and taste improves. A major consideration is a reduced risk of developing emphysema and osteoporosis.

Over a period of time, from two weeks to three months, your circulation will improve significantly. Smokers tend to feel colder than nonsmokers do in the same temperatures. You'll find that walking and other exercise gets easier as your lung function improves. Coaches were among the first people to urge athletes to quit, even before doctors did, because they saw how smoking saps performance. Pay attention to the improvements in your health and remind yourself that these are the rewards for the discomforts you've been feeling, because, let's face the facts, quitting isn't easy or pleasant. But I can tell you this: it's better than a heart attack. I've been there. I know.

In the coming months, you'll feel better and better. You'll cough less and less. Sinus congestion diminishes. You'll feel more energy and less fatigue. Notice when you climb a flight of stairs that you're not as short of breath.

By the end of the first nonsmoking year, your risk of developing heart disease is down to half that of a smoker. After five to fifteen years, the chances of your suffering a stroke are cut to those of people who have never smoked. When you celebrate your tenth anniversary of quitting, remember that your risk of developing lung cancer is half that of smokers. You'll also improve your odds against getting ulcers and a wide variety of other cancers.

In fifteen years, your risk of heart disease is no different from that of men and women who never smoked a cigarette. Your expected life span will be about the same as well.

All these statistics were part of the U.S. Surgeon General's report in 1990. I can add from personal experience and from what I've learned from others that you'll sleep more soundly, wake more rested, have more energy, and just feel better in general.

Withdrawal Symptoms

Why is it so difficult to quit? Smoking is far more than a bad habit like squeezing the toothpaste in the middle of the tube. You have both a powerful psychological pattern and a true chemical addiction that's as strong as being hooked on heroin or cocaine. Nonsmokers just don't understand that, and neither did the medical community until fairly recently. Former heroin addicts have told me that quitting that drug was *easier* than quitting cigarettes.

Here's something to think about. A heavily addicted drug addict might shoot up three or four times a day. If you smoke a pack a day, you're getting a fix twenty times daily. I did two packs of Marlboros a day at my point of deepest addiction. So I needed *forty fixes each and every day*! Modern medical imaging systems allow scientists to look at the brain before and after either a hit of a drug or a puff from a cigarette. The pictures look the same. In technical terms, dopamine receptor sites in the brain crave the next wave of satisfaction.

This is something that smokers do not realize. I know I didn't. I looked forward to having the next cigarette. I said I enjoyed that cigarette. That was especially true when I had to go without a smoke for a longer than average time, as when at a movie or in church. Ah, that cigarette I craved tasted so good! But the reality is far different from enjoying a fine piece of chocolate or the scent of the Christmas tree when it first goes up in December.

In truth, you're not really enjoying the taste of the cigarette. You're enjoying the freedom from the craving that's emanated from your brain and affected your entire body. After having, say, that piece of chocolate, do you have a strong craving for more an hour or so later? A craving so demanding that you'd go to the trash can to find the candy wrapping and lick it to get a little taste? The way I know you do when you're out of cigarettes in the middle of the night and you light up a burned butt from the ashtray? There's no comparison. Craving a cigarette is a demonstration of addiction, not appreciation.

The source of that addiction is nicotine. Try to switch to a light cigarette and you'll simply smoke more to get the amount of nicotine you now need. Not want, need. The tobacco companies have known that for decades and they've made sure that cigarettes deliver the amount of nicotine a smoker craves. Cigarettes truly are delivery systems for nicotine, a substance just as addictive as any other drug.

The bad news is that you'll start experiencing nicotine withdrawal symptoms at the exact moment when you'd normally light your next cigarette. The first of those symptoms will be edginess, restlessness, irritability, and a general frustration that might even make you prowl the room like a caged tiger. You might have trouble concentrating; that was particularly difficult for me at the typewriter. Some people experience dizziness during the first day or two. Others go into a bit of depression, might have trouble sleeping, or find themselves feeling hungry all the time. I'll talk about the weight issue later.

At the beginning, there's only one way to get rid of all those symptoms instantly: light another cigarette. Don't do it. The worst symptoms occur during the first two or three days of withdrawal. Then, after that, the cravings and the withdrawal symptoms will gradually decrease. The good news is that typically after just two or three weeks, your body is free of nicotine addiction. That is to say, those receptor sites in the brain will no longer be screaming for you to light another butt.

Here's a radical concept. Instead of viewing the withdrawal symptoms as painful and horrible and of no value, make an active, conscious effort to accept each craving as a part of the learning curve. When the urge to light up becomes almost unbearable, *think* about how that craving will pass and how such desires are becoming fewer and further between. Moreover, think about that craving, though unquestionably painful, as a small price to pay for the freedom you're fighting for. That's right, you've become a freedom fighter, battling an addiction that has killed millions but that has been beaten by millions more. Notice that today you have had fewer cravings than yesterday. Tomorrow there will be fewer still. You're able to deal with and beat back that craving more effectively with each passing day. If you're a religious person, by all means ask for divine assistance. Pray to get through that compelling desire. Or think intensively about the many reasons you want to quit. Work your way through each wave of craving by taking an active role: go take a walk for a few minutes; maybe this is the time to shine your shoes, empty the trash, or do a few sit-ups or whatever can take your mind off the moment. Always remember that the physical withdrawal symptoms will last, at most, only a few weeks.

Unfortunately, there is also the psychological addiction, far worse than the word *habit* implies. The reason is very simple. We smokers learned to smoke a cigarette with everything from a phone call to a cup of coffee to lovemaking. These associations are difficult to break. We literally have to learn to *not* smoke at each and every one of those cues. The more cigarettes one smokes during a typical day, over the course of a week or more, the greater the number of cues.

While that may seem enormously difficult at first, it's also a way to break the quitting process down into reasonable bites. First, decide what your most frequent, most urgent cues are. Yours will be different from mine. A college roommate of mine always smoked a cigarette while sitting on the toilet in the morning. After he quit, that daily bowel movement brought urges to light up. Spend a little time thinking about your strongest associations. Jot these down on a piece of paper. Then think about what you can do to break each particular habit, one at a time.

Here are a few suggestions:

- Instead of having a cup of coffee during the morning and the afternoon break, go for a ten-minute walk.
- Rather than lingering at the dinner table after a meal, immediately get up and start cleaning off the dishes and the utensils.
- Replace your cigarette pack with a tin of sour candies or mints in your pocket so that you'll have something to reach for when the phone rings or an office meeting begins. A bartender I knew kept a pocketful of swizzle sticks to chew during the day.

As time goes on, and the cravings and desires pass, you'll be able to live through each and every one of those cues without the cigarettes and their temporary replacements and diversions. But don't be surprised if, even months or years later, something signals an urge to light a cigarette.

I remember one evening when my wife, Dawn, and I were having a drink at one of the few bars in Los Angeles with a commanding view of the city. It's called the SkyBar. Seated at a table next to the floor-to-ceiling window and gazing out at the sparkling lights beneath us, I had this powerful desire to have a cigarette. That was about six years after I'd quit smoking, and I thought the habit was completely broken. So what was going on?

In Chicago, where Dawn and I had lived before moving west to California, we enjoyed countless evenings in just such a setting. We were both smokers at the time. The pleasures of those evenings and smoking were strongly linked. It had been years since our days in high-rise apartments, restaurants, and bars in the Windy City. That view from the SkyBar window sparked my memories and those cravings for a cigarette. I had not yet learned to enjoy such moments without lighting up. So that evening I learned to enjoy that atmosphere without smoking. In a few minutes, the craving was gone and Dawn and I had a good laugh over it. I never again had that desire strike in similar circumstances.

When I quit, I tried not to smoke one day at a time. I recommend that you do the same. Don't try to imagine not smoking for the rest of your life. That's too much to handle at once.

As each day went by, the length of time that the craving persisted became shorter. A few things definitely helped. Getting up from a chair and walking, even just across the room. Taking a deep breath, and concentrating on breathing to take my mind off the craving. Having a sip of water. Playing a game of solitaire to keep my hands busy. Going to movie theaters and other places where smoking was prohibited.

Smoking Cessation Aids

Although the psychological addiction takes longer to deal with, it isn't as dramatic or as traumatic as withdrawal from nicotine. Fortunately, there are several aids to wean smokers gradually off nicotine. They work better for some men and women than for others, but you owe it to yourself to give them a try to improve your chances of success. While many people quit without using those aids, anyone who gives in to lighting up again does so primarily owing to the strength of that nicotine addiction and craving.

Nicotine replacement in the form of patches, gum, lozenges, inhalers, and sprays is a way of tapering off the amount of nicotine your body needs on a daily basis to let you maintain a sense of equilibrium and comfort. These aids greatly reduce withdrawal symptoms. Pregnant women and people with existing heart disease should speak with a physician before using methods of nicotine replacement.

Studies have shown that nicotine replacement greatly improves one's chances of quitting successfully. Combining that with a support group of some kind can double the odds of success. More about those support groups later.

If you're going to use one of those aids, it's best to do so from the very start, rather than waiting until the withdrawal symptoms become intolerable. You need all the help you can get. I wish those aids had been around in 1979!

For details concerning the various nicotine-replacement aids, including how best to use them and potential side effects, visit www.cancer.org or one of the other sources of information I've provided at the end of this chapter. You may also want to discuss their use with your physician.

Prescription Drugs

Almost everyone who quits smoking goes through a period of significant stress. Irritability, restlessness, inability to concentrate on one's work, and other symptoms are pretty common. Adding everyday stress and strains to this may undermine one's success in quitting.

The drug bupropion, sold as Wellbutrin SR and Zyban, is a prescription-only antidepressant that has been successfully used to help smokers quit. It targets the pleasure centers of the brain. Again, talk with your doctor about possibly getting a prescription to help you cope with the emotional components of quitting.

The latest drug, Chantix (varenicline), was approved by the FDA in May 2006. It appears to reduce nicotine craving by blocking the effect of the nicotine on the brain. Clinical testing showed much better short- and long-term rates of quitting in people taking Chantix than in subjects taking either bupropion or a placebo, but there was a rather high rate of nausea as a side effect. Talk with your doctor about whether either of these drugs might be right for you. Three reports on Chantix were published in the July 5, 2006, issue of the *Journal of the American Medical Association*.

In addition to these drugs, there are other ways of dealing with stress, while you attempt to quit smoking and at other times as well. Regular exercise is one of the best coping tools. Rigorous physical activity, in fact, causes the brain to release the body's natural relaxants, the beta-endorphins, which can have a truly potent soothing effect. Many of us who are hooked on exercise really enjoy the feeling that a good workout can provide. The effects last for hours, well into the day or evening. For more approaches to stress control, see chapter 7, "Reduce Your Stress."

Support Groups and Other Helpers

The best support while you're trying to quit smoking should come from your family, friends, and coworkers. When you decide to quit, tell all of them. Many will be former smokers, familiar with the difficulties of quitting. They'll remember how they were grumpy and irritable during the withdrawal period. Explain to people who have never smoked that your grouchiness and occasional nastiness have nothing to do with them, and ask them to be as understanding as possible.

In addition, there are both nonprofit and for-profit organizations that can help you get over this hurdle in your life. The best of these groups will include either individual or group counseling. Choose a support group that will give intense assistance in terms of offering more or longer sessions or both. There are definite similarities here with alcoholic treatment centers. In fact, one group is called Nicotine Anonymous. You'll want to have sessions that are at least twenty to thirty minutes long each time, frequently throughout the week, for at least two to three weeks.

For help in finding and choosing a support group, contact your local American Cancer Society, American Lung Association, American Heart Association, or your physician or local hospital.

Hypnosis and acupuncture are rather controversial among health authorities. Some of them see potential benefit and recommend that smokers give these methods a try. Others feel that there is no scientific evidence that either one really works. Certainly, you can find former smokers who swear by one or the other. If you've tried quitting again and again without success, you might want to give one or both a try.

Smoking and Weight Gain

Decades ago, tobacco companies advertised their deadly products as a way to lose and maintain weight. Indeed, the sad fact is that people who quit smoking often do gain weight. That's more the case for women than for men, although both are likely to put on a few pounds while shedding the cigarette habit.

Don't let the prospect of weight gain weaken your resolve to stop smoking cigarettes. Certainly, the health benefits of quitting far outbalance the ill effects of slight weight gain. Once you're comfortable in your life as a nonsmoker, you can deal with getting rid of the pounds you put on during that life-saving effort.

Yet there are definitely ways you can, at the very least, limit the amount of weight you will gain. Follow a healthy diet that's low in fat, nutrient-poor carbohydrates, and calories. When choosing snacks and "nibbles" to replace cigarettes throughout the day, opt for those lowest in calories, such as pretzels, popcorn, sugar-free hard candies, carrot sticks, celery stalks, and the like. And be certain to engage in some physical activity each and every day.

Quid pro quo is a term often used in the practice of law to indicate a trade-off, literally translated as "this for that." Offer yourself a reward for quitting those cigarettes. Do a calculation of how much money you spend daily, weekly, monthly, and yearly to smoke. You'll probably be shocked at the high number you come up with, even though you're aware that it's been an expensive habit. Then decide what you'd rather do with the money you'll save.

Start a "quitter's bank" and put the money you've saved each week into a coffee can or a pickle jar. Keep that money separate from your ordinary budget, the one that pays for necessities. Maybe you'll have enough money to buy a piece of jewelry. Or perhaps you'd prefer a weekend getaway with your spouse or a friend. It's your choice, and you deserve it!

Helping a Smoker Quit

If your friend or loved one has decided to quit, you can and will play an important role in his or her success or failure. You might, for example, be tempted to tell that person to light up a cigarette just to end the grumpiness. That's happened more than once in lots and lots of families. Conversely, you don't want to tell him or her how to quit, even if it's a trick you found valuable when you quit a while back. This isn't the time to offer advice. It won't be taken very well.

But there's a lot you can do to ensure success. Quitting smoking is a major decision and a difficult task. Congratulate the person for taking that first step. Offer to help in any way you can, even if that means staying out of sight as much as possible! My wife says to this day that she never would have been able to quit if I hadn't taken the kids away for a week's fishing. She just wanted to be left alone.

The quitter is going to be grumpy, grouchy, irritable, nasty, insulting, and just plain miserable to be with. That goes with the territory for everyone but a saint, and there aren't too many of them around! Accept the trade-off of future good health and an environment free of smoke, ashtrays, and stink. Assuming that he or she was lovable before trying to quit, he or she will be so again in just two or three weeks.

If someone quits smoking, that's taking a big step toward improved health, which includes gaining control of his or her blood pressure and reducing the risk of having a heart attack or a stroke. Without going over the top about it, give the person frequent congratulations. Take note of the first cigarette-free week and subsequent landmarks.

Help to keep the quitter's mind off smoking. Suggest a movie. Or a game of cards. Or a walk in the woods or along the beach.

Remember that it's just a matter of time, and try to help the time pass a bit faster during the cessation process. That person is worth it.

Quitting cigarettes was one of the most difficult things I have done in my life. It also helped to save my life. I wish you the same success.

There's a lot of useful information available on the Internet for people who want to quit smoking cigarettes.

American Cancer Society
www.cancer.org

American Heart Association & American Stroke Association
www.amhrt.org
www.strokeassociation.org

American Lung Association
www.lungusa.org

Centers for Disease Control and Prevention
Office on Smoking and Health
www.cdc.gov/tobacco

National Cancer Institute
www.cancer.gov

Nicotine Anonymous
www.nicotine-anonymous.org

Smokefree.gov (including information on state Quitlines)
www.smokefree.gov

Smoking Cessation Leadership Center
http://smokingcessationleadership.ucsf.edu

9

Balance Your Electrolytes: Sodium, Potassium, Calcium, and Magnesium

We've all heard the same advice: cut back on salt and sodium in our diets. That advice has been around so long, in fact, that most people just accept it at face value, assuming that taking the salt shaker off the dinner table will cause their blood pressure to come down and their hearts to get healthier. Well, it's just not that simple. We have to take sodium restriction recommendations with the proverbial grain of salt.

Without my going into a lot of scientific details that you really don't need to know, suffice it to say that sodium is one of four electrolytes—the others are calcium, magnesium, and potassium—needed by the body to achieve its daily functions. Every time the heart beats or the muscles contract, electrolytes come into play. Without the proper combination, the heart would stop beating and muscles would go either rigid or flaccid. Messages pass through our nervous systems as sodium enters a nerve cell and potassium exits. After the message is transmitted, sodium leaves the cell. Without that so-called sodium-potassium pump, our bodies would pretty much shut down. Similarly, we can't do without calcium and magnesium, either.

The body performs an elaborate and exquisite balancing act to keep electrolytes working together to maintain body functions, including blood pressure. We can do a lot to help that vital balancing act.

Salt makes our foods taste better, and most of us living in Western civilizations consume too much of it. No question about that. We'd get all the sodium we need from just one daily teaspoon of salt, sodium chloride. But we like to put it into the water before boiling potatoes or making pasta, and we sprinkle on more when we sit down to eat. In addition, 75 percent of the sodium in our diets comes from processed foods that contain not only sodium chloride but also a whole family of sodium compounds to make those foods taste good and make them last longer on supermarket shelves and in our pantries, bread boxes, and refrigerators.

The other electrolytes, unfortunately, don't taste as good. We don't sprinkle potassium chloride on our popcorn or put it on the rims of margarita glasses, although we might want to get into the habit of consuming more potassium, as well as more calcium and magnesium.

Should Everyone Restrict Salt and Sodium?

Heart authorities in the United States, the United Kingdom, Australia, and just about everywhere else urge citizens to cut back, way back, on salt and sodium consumption. For many people, this can help them to control hypertension. That's especially true for blacks and older men and women, all of whom are more salt sensitive than others. About 25 to 50 percent, perhaps more, of people with hypertension—not necessarily mildly elevated blood pressure—are sodium sensitive. Blacks have a higher rate of sodium sensitivity, but that leaves a lot of men and women who are not.

There's no doubt that genetics play a major role in how the body deals with sodium. The way our kidneys handle salt and sodium makes the difference. Let's look at a study done with rats in the laboratory that are bred to be either sodium sensitive or sodium resistant. The blood pressure of sensitive rats goes up quickly when they're fed a diet high in sodium. But the blood pressure of sodium-resistant rats is not affected. When the kidney from a sodium-resistant rat is transplanted to a sodium-sensitive rat, blood pressure goes down. Conversely, blood pressure goes up in sodium-resistant rats given a sodium-sensitive kidney.

In a nutshell, salt and other sodium compounds are involved in a chemical sequence initiated in the kidneys that ends with the production of a substance, angiotensin, that raises blood pressure. In fact, some of the blood pressure drugs that doctors prescribe block the action of that angiotensin. The more sensitive one is to sodium, the more angiotensin gets made in the kidney, the more sodium is stored in the body, and the more water is retained in the body's tissues. All of this raises blood pressure.

The antisalt zealots like to point to the famous International Intersalt Study, the most comprehensive effort undertaken in this field thus far. Researchers looked at blood pressure and sodium intake in thirty-two countries. For the most part, the results revealed few links between sodium intake and hypertension in people around the world. That said, however, people in countries that had extremely high salt intake tended to have higher levels of blood pressure, while individuals with very little salt in their diets had lower levels. But these are the extremes. For most people in most countries, there was little association between salt and sodium consumption and blood pressure. And, paradoxically, people in Thailand who traditionally eat very salty diets had relatively low blood pressure levels.

Here's the basic truth. Take a person with normal blood pressure, feed him or her excessive amounts of salt, and blood pressure will go up. Bring that salt intake back down and blood pressure goes down along with it. That physiological fact was even demonstrated in chimpanzees, animals that are pretty similar to us in many ways. But, again, we're talking about extremes. These and other findings suggest that unless sodium is very severely limited, most people will not see any improvement. Any drop in blood pressure, on average, will be clinically insignificant. Just for the heck of it, let's look a little closer at that chimp study, done by Australian scientists in Gabon, Africa.

Chimpanzees naturally consume a diet consisting mostly of fruit and vegetable matter. Half the chimps in the study were given a liquid that provided up to 15 grams of salt daily, a massive amount. After twenty months on the salt-laced diet, seven of the thirteen chimps showed a big increase in both systolic and diastolic blood pressure. But three chimps showed no change at all and three didn't drink all the salt solution. Still, the conclusion was that salt raises blood pressure.

Bear in mind that data in all such studies reflect averages. Even in a population where salt intake is very high, only some individuals will show a rise in blood pressure. The majority will have normal blood pressure, even if they consume the same amount of salt that the others do. But when people who play with statistics take those data and crunch them all together, they can find *on average* that reduced salt or sodium intake lowers blood pressure. Statistics may show, to exaggerate my point just a bit, that the average family has 2.2 children, but I've yet to see a cradle or a stroller containing 0.2 child! Forget those averages; let's talk instead about real, individual men and women.

Let's look at just one of the many studies done with real human subjects. For three years, 841 men and women were observed for the blood pressure-lowering effects of diet. Some people restricted sodium, some cut back on calories, and others reduced both sodium and calories. The group with the greatest drop in blood pressure was that which reduced calories. People cutting back on sodium alone showed very little difference.

Within those groups, however, were men and women who were very sensitive to sodium. Salt or sodium sensitivity is a very real thing. Researchers are now trying to develop a test for such sensitivity so that physicians can know which patients need sodium restriction and which do not, rather than prescribing it for everyone. That test is still in the future, but the zealots say we don't need such a test because if everyone greatly restricted sodium intake, some people would benefit and society would be the better for it. Maybe some day we'll have that sensitivity test, and maybe not. In the meantime, we do know that African Americans, older individuals, people who are overweight, and those who consume little dietary fiber are more likely to be sensitive.

In 2002, the *British Medical Journal* published a review of eleven trials of interventions aimed at reducing dietary salt intake. Tens of thousands of subjects were involved, with and without hypertension. Follow-up ranged from six months to seven years, comparing the blood pressure reductions of people following the advice of salt restriction with those in the control groups, people not given that advice. The average difference was a mere 1.1 mm Hg systolic blood pressure and 0.6 mm Hg diastolic.

In a commentary in the publication *Journal Watch*, the reviewing physician, Keith Marton, M.D., wrote that "These interventions were highly restrictive and, as such, unlikely to be useful in primary care. Thus, the mild effect of dietary salt restriction on BP hardly seems worth the effort, especially given the apparent lack of significant effect on overall health."

But Dr. Marton also noted that "these results do not rule out the possibility that an individual patient occasionally will have a more substantial response to salt restriction." Such individuals are most likely to be African American, overweight, older, and hypertensive, since these men and women are more often salt sensitive. And data reported in 2005 from the University of Miami in Florida indicate that women may become more salt sensitive as they enter their postmenopausal years.

How can you tell whether restricting your sodium intake will lower your blood pressure? Experiment. Try testing yourself. Measure your blood pressure for a few days in a row. Cut back on processed foods, don't add salt when cooking, and put the salt shaker away. Do that for a few weeks and retest your blood pressure. See whether you benefit. If so, terrific. If not, there are other ways of lowering blood pressure.

It may even be possible that a low-salt diet can do more harm than good. Dr. Brent Egan, then at the Medical College of Wisconsin in Milwaukee, found that a low-salt diet will not reduce blood pressure in 50 percent of people with higher-than-normal blood pressure and in 80 percent of individuals with more normal blood pressure. In fact, for some people, salt restriction may actually result in higher blood pressure!

Even more disturbing was a study linking low sodium consumption with an increase in heart attack risk. Working with hypertensive men at the Albert Einstein College of Medicine in New York City, Dr. Michael Alderman detected an unexpectedly high incidence of heart attacks in men who had low amounts of salt in their urine, reflecting their dietary restrictions. The study followed nearly two thousand men for almost four years. More than four times as many heart attacks occurred in men with the lowest amounts of sodium in their urine compared with men who had the highest amounts of urinary sodium.

Dr. Alderman also studied more than a thousand hypertensive women, but only nine of them suffered heart attacks during the study period, too small a number to draw any conclusions. Among the men, there were forty-six heart attacks.

These data don't mean that everyone should rush out and start gobbling salt. The patients involved had significant hypertension and other factors to consider. But the findings do cast a big shadow on blanket recommendations that everyone should severely restrict his or her sodium consumption.

So what are doctors and their patients to do? Dr. Egan takes a very practical approach with his own patients. He has them monitor their blood pressure for a week before starting a low-salt diet in order to establish a baseline. Then they keep track of their pressure after cutting back on salt. If there is no reduction in blood pressure after one to two months, Dr. Egan tells them to discontinue salt restriction. After all, why follow a prescription that doesn't work, any more than a physician would have a patient continue to take a drug that didn't achieve the desired effect?

As the old saying goes, all things in moderation. The same advice should be given regarding salt and sodium intake. Practically all of us in the United States and other affluent countries around the world consume way too much salt. Even if becoming more moderate doesn't lower our blood pressure, there are other benefits, including an easing of the burden on the kidneys and a lessening of water retention. Most of the weight loss when you start a diet comes from water loss. Cut back—reasonably—on salt and sodium-rich foods and that water and weight loss can be permanent. Moderation, not restriction.

Most of the sodium in the American diet comes from processed foods, such as canned vegetables and soups and snack foods, as well as from fast foods. Simply cutting back on those foods will slash your sodium intake enormously. Instead of canned vegetables, use frozen veggies, which are actually less expensive, have no sodium, and taste a lot better. Of course, fresh is even better, but nothing beats the convenience of frozen. Opt for low-sodium versions of chicken broth. Start reading those Nutrition Facts labels and choose foods that are lower in sodium. Rather than going for the usual deep-fried fast foods, try a sandwich shop such as Subway, Quiznos, or Blimpie or stop in at a supermarket, most of which have pre-made sandwiches in the deli department.

My wife and I enjoyed a little weekend getaway at a Japanese hotel in Los Angeles that featured an authentic Japanese lifestyle. This included the room, the grounds, a plunge pool and hot baths, shiatsu massage, and traditional foods for breakfast, lunch, and dinner. Japanese foods are notorious for their high salt content. By the end of the weekend, we couldn't remove the rings from our water-swollen fingers. Wow, what a dramatic demonstration of excess consumption! It's no surprise that the Japanese suffer a high rate of hypertension and strokes.

So how can we cut back and still enjoy our foods? First of all, understand that we have become habituated to a high-salt diet. After two to three weeks, the urge to salt everything on the plate passes, and after a couple of months you begin to enjoy the natural flavors of foods and you find that the kinds of foods you previously consumed taste overly salty.

Even the water we drink contains some sodium but only about 1 percent of our total consumption. Obviously, we don't want to restrict our water drinking. Next, foods in their natural state, even fruits and vegetables and, more notably, dairy foods, provide about 12 percent of our salt intake. Surely, we don't want to eliminate any of those healthy foods. The salt shaker on the table adds 6 percent and cooking contributes 5 percent. So where does most of our salt and sodium come from? A whopping 75 to 77 percent is in processed, manufactured, and packaged foods and meals eaten in fast-food restaurants. That's where we need to cut back. But we want to do so selectively.

Bread is made with salt, even though it doesn't taste salty. Try eating low-salt or salt-free bread and you're in for a horrible experience. The stuff tastes like cardboard, with no flavor whatsoever. Try to make those kinds of changes, and you're doomed to failure.

Instead, start with baby steps. If a recipe calls for 28 ounces of canned tomatoes, use a 14-ounce can of ordinary tomatoes and another 14-ounce can of no-salt-added tomatoes. You eliminate half the salt and virtually none of the flavor. Use the same approach for most other canned and processed foods. As time goes by, and your taste buds change, you'll be able to switch to more low-salt foods. It's pretty easy to see how much sodium is in a given processed food, since the quantity per serving is listed on all labels.

Staying away from fast-food restaurants is healthy for many reasons beyond salt reduction. You'll also slash your consumption of total, saturated, and trans fats, as well as calories. The United States has made some very fine contributions to the world, but fast-food restaurants are not among them. In 2005, I was saddened during a month-long trip to China to see streets lined with McDonald's, Pizza Huts, and KFC restaurants. The Chinese love KFC the most, savoring deep-fried chicken skin. Sound disgusting? Remember that Peking duck feasts offer slices of the skin with very little meat; most of the carcass is discarded.

I realize that my next suggestion will sound almost revolutionary, if not completely out of the realm of reason and practicality. Try cooking and eating more at home, enjoying homemade foods. Again, start with baby steps of perhaps one extra homemade meal per week. I think some of my recipe suggestions at the end of this book will make your mouth water and will tempt you to try to prepare those dishes, many if not most of which are designed to lower blood pressure—not because of what they don't contain but because of what they do, in keeping with a Mediterranean diet. More about that later.

Right now, we're talking about sodium and don't forget those other electrolytes. It's difficult, I believe, to accurately keep track of the actual amount of salt or sodium we eat daily. I think that merely following the previous suggestions to whatever extent you are willing to will be adequate for the average person, especially if extreme sodium restriction is not mandatory, as might be the case for someone with severe hypertension, the sort of patient who would often be prescribed a minimum of two and up to five different drugs to control his or her blood pressure. For the record, the recommended amount of sodium for men and women is 1,500 mg in the United States. That's a little less than about one teaspoonful. Again, other than perhaps some very diligent dietitians, I doubt that many individuals have any idea as to how much salt or sodium they consume daily, or what it would mean to cut back to suggested levels. That's why I put forth my ideas on how to rather painlessly reduce intake in the previous paragraphs. So what can we do beyond trying a reasonable, moderate sodium cutback?

Do you use a water softener? You might be getting a lot of sodium from the water you're drinking. That could be particularly important if you're sodium sensitive. Have an unsoftened water line for drinking and cooking purposes. Water-softening systems that use potassium- rather than sodium-based softening agents might be a good idea, giving you an additional source of that mineral, another electrolyte in the balancing act—unless your physician has advised you to limit potassium because you have problems with your kidney function.

It is my fervent belief that cutting back on salt and sodium offers just a small, though useful, start to improving our blood pressure status. Probably far more important is making a real effort to increase the other electrolytes: calcium, magnesium, and potassium. I think that most of the benefit in switching from salt to a salt substitute at the dinner table or for food preparation comes not from cutting back on the sodium chloride but, rather, from increasing our consumption of potassium chloride.

Potassium and Blood Pressure

Most national health authorities now recommend increased potassium consumption, along with their advice to cut back on sodium. That's true for the U.S. Dietary Guidelines Advisory Committee; the National Academy of Sciences' Food and Nutrition Board; the National Heart, Lung, and Blood Institute of the National Institutes of Health; the American Heart Association; Health Canada; and the Australian Heart Foundation. The reason for this unanimity is simple: the science just can't be denied. Potassium is a chemical element that helps to maintain normal functioning of muscles, the heart, and the nervous system. Potassium is a major regulator of blood pressure.

Too much sodium in the body signals the kidneys to raise blood pressure. Too little potassium has the same effect. It's the yin and yang of the body's balance. And most Americans consume too little potassium.

In 1991, University of Pennsylvania researchers found that just ten days of potassium restriction resulted in rises in blood pressure, whether one had normal or elevated blood pressure to begin with. A twelve-year study of California adults suggested that high potassium intake protects against stroke, the worst result of hypertension. For men in that study, those with low potassium intake had 2.6 times more stroke risk than did men with high consumption of potassium-rich foods. For women, low intake multiplied the risk by nearly five times.

Potassium restriction was also associated with sodium retention and with calcium depletion in various studies. The converse is also true, giving one good explanation as to why potassium works so well. The mineral causes the body to excrete more sodium in the urine, the same mode of action achieved with antihypertensive drugs called thiazide diuretics. Potassium seems to correct salt sensitivity as well.

In 1994, doctors at Johns Hopkins Hospital in Baltimore, Maryland, investigated the potential of adding potassium to the diet. They gave potassium supplements to one group of African Americans known to have a high incidence of salt sensitivity and hypertension and a placebo to a similar group. Both groups had what would be termed high normal blood pressure or prehypertension, 125/77 in one and 127/78 in the other.

At the end of just three weeks, systolic blood pressure had dropped an average of 6.9 points in people taking the potassium supplements, and diastolic readings tumbled by 2.5 points. That's a lot of improvement for little effort.

More recently, British researchers gave half of a group of sixty-nine healthy volunteers potassium supplements three times daily, providing the amount of the mineral found in five servings of fruits and vegetables. The other volunteers got a placebo. At the end of the six-week trial, people getting the potassium enjoyed a decline in systolic blood pressure of 7.60 mm Hg and a drop of 6.46 mm Hg in diastolic blood pressure. Improvement occurred gradually over the six-week period of time.

Can making a little change like using a salt substitute to provide extra potassium lengthen your life? A study from Taiwan provides a very promising answer. About two thousand men in a Taiwanese retirement home were given food prepared with either regular salt or a salt substitute that was half sodium chloride and half potassium chloride. During the relatively short period of just thirty months, men who got the salt substitute were 40 percent less likely to die from cardiovascular disease.

Was it because of the reduction in sodium? Perhaps that was part of it, but one of the researchers in the study published in the June 2006 issue of the *American Journal of Clinical Nutrition* believes it was more likely due to the increased potassium.

Again, there's no doubt in the scientific and medical communities that potassium is one answer to the blood pressure problems in Western countries around the world.

There are additional benefits from making sure your diet is rich in potassium. The mineral helps to prevent kidney stones and heartbeat disturbances called arrhythmias. It also keeps bones strong by neutralizing acids in the bloodstream that leach calcium from bone.

Paleontologists studying the eating habits of our early ancestors have universally found that their diet was low in sodium and high in potassium. They ate a lot of very lean meat whenever they could get it and relied heavily on fruits and vegetables. Conversely, our modern diet is high in sodium and low in potassium, since we eat sodium-rich processed foods and fewer fruits and veggies.

Sadly, except for vegetarians—who still might consume too much sodium, by the way—most of us get too little potassium in our diets because we just don't eat enough fruits and vegetables. That's been shown to be the case in the United States, Canada, the United Kingdom, Australia, and Europe. Typically, the most frequently eaten vegetable is French-fried potatoes or potato chips or crisps.

So, how much potassium should we shoot for? Recommendations call for at least 4.7 grams daily to lower blood pressure, blunt the effects of salt, reduce the risk of kidney stones and bone loss, and stabilize heartbeat. Round that off to 5 grams. Although you shouldn't go hog wild by going overboard with potassium supplements and potassium-containing salt substitutes, many, if not most, authorities would agree that you just can't consume too much of this "miracle" mineral.

Ideally, the ratio of potassium to sodium in our diet should be about five to one. But the typical American, and for that matter Western, diet provides almost exactly the opposite! The solution is obvious: cut back on salt and sodium where you'll miss them least, as in canned vegetables and other processed foods and fast foods, and make a conscious effort to boost your potassium consumption.

Here's just one example of how you might do that in your life. One cup of regular chicken broth contains a whopping 960 mg of sodium; replace that with reduced-sodium broth or, better yet, salt-free chicken broth. That day, enjoy a one-cup serving of sweet potato to add 950 mg of potassium. By cutting the sodium and boosting the potassium, in this instance, you've completely reversed the potassium/sodium ratio in the right direction.

Potassium is really easy to get just by paying a little more attention to our diets. Because the health benefits of potassium are now being proclaimed, many food companies are listing the amount of the mineral on food labels when certain foods offer a significant contribution. Raw foods, of course, don't carry nutrition information labels, so here's a chart of some of the best sources of potassium.

Food	Amount	Potassium (mg)
Fruits and Vegetables		
Sweet potato	1 cup	950
Honeydew melon	¼ melon	940
Acorn squash	1 cup	900
Potato (baked)	1 medium	844
Avocado	½ medium	680
Dried figs	5 whole	666
Prunes	10 medium	626
Dates	10 whole	541
Tomato puree	½ cup	525
Dried apricots	10 halves	482
Banana	1 medium	451
Cantaloupe	1 cup	450
Orange juice	1 cup	450
Winter squash	½ cup	445
Raisins	½ cup	375
Lima beans	½ cup	370
Mango	1 medium	323
Orange	1 medium	250
Strawberries	1 cup	247
Meats		
Broiled lean beef	3½ ounces	426
Lamb sirloin	3½ ounces	183
Broiled pork loin	3½ ounces	375
Seasonings		
Cream of tartar	1 teaspoon	495
Salt Substitutes		
Morton light salt	1 teaspoon	1,500
Morton salt substitute	1 teaspoon	2,800
No Salt	1 teaspoon	2,500

Surely, in that listing, there must be some foods that start your mouth watering! Why not add some of them to your shopping list right now? And be sure to include some dried fruits, such as apricots and raisins that you can keep in the car, your purse, or the office for handy, healthy snacks. Shoot for a potassium intake of at least 3,500 mg daily, ideally 4,700 mg (4.7 grams/120 mmol).

Notice that the salt substitutes provide a whopping amount of potassium, using potassium chloride instead of sodium chloride. Just replacing the salt shaker with one of those substitutes, or using both intermittently, will help to boost your potassium intake and lower your blood pressure. Don't like the taste? Add some to foods as they're cooking and you won't even notice. Add a teaspoon of salt substitute to water when you cook pasta and vegetables. Stir it into soups and stews. Blend it in with other ingredients when you make a meatloaf or other dishes. Then use just a tiny sprinkle of regular table salt when you eat.

Forget the potassium supplement tablets that are available in many stores and pharmacies. On a bottle that I checked, one potassium gluconate tablet is listed as containing 550 mg. But read the information on the back label and you'll learn, as I did, that the tablet actually contains only 90 mg of actual potassium. You can get five times as much from a glass of orange juice.

Adding extra potassium to the diet is a great idea for practically everyone who wants to lower his or her blood pressure, but there are exceptions. Don't do so if you have kidney problems or if you are currently taking the antihypertensive drugs called ACE inhibitors. If you have any doubts, talk with your doctor about the advantages and disadvantages of the potassium boost.

Calcium and Blood Pressure

Dr. David McCarron of the Oregon Health Sciences University in Portland pioneered the research showing that insufficient calcium in the diet could be as important, or even more so, than consuming too much sodium. Additional studies have corroborated his initial findings.

In a project at Johns Hopkins University in Baltimore, researchers found that twenty-three women who took 1.5 grams or 2 grams of calcium carbonate supplements daily throughout pregnancy decreased their diastolic blood pressure by 4 to 7 mm Hg. The higher calcium dosage yielded the more dramatic blood pressure improvements. Results were the same in both white and black women.

The research has been international. Dutch investigators reported lowering blood pressure with calcium supplements. One gram daily dropped diastolic blood pressure by 3.1 mm Hg in just six weeks. In one of the largest studies of its kind, California medical scientists found that increasing daily calcium intake by 1 gram lowered the risk of high blood pressure by 12 percent on average for the 6,634 men and women participating. Benefits are greater for certain individuals. People under forty have 25 percent less risk per gram of calcium. Lean men and women demonstrate an 18 percent risk reduction. Individuals drinking less than one alcoholic beverage per day get a 16 percent cut in hypertension risk per calcium gram consumed.

How does calcium work its wonders on blood pressure? This gets a bit technical. The mineral reduces the concentration of parathyroid hormone in the blood; that hormone regulates calcium metabolism. In turn, that might lower calcium concentrations in the body's cells and slow the calcium from entering the arteries. Calcium in the arteries affects the tone of the vessels, thus potentially leading to higher blood pressure as the arteries stiffen.

Calcium supplements that a woman takes during pregnancy may leave a lasting benefit by lowering her child's blood pressure. Toddlers whose mothers took prenatal calcium supplements had lower blood pressure levels than did those whose mothers did not. According to the lead investigator of that study in Oregon, such calcium intake may help to "program" fetal blood pressure, possibly with effects that last into adulthood.

View supplements as just that: an adjunct to, not a replacement for, dietary calcium. Nonfat and low-fat dairy foods, with the exception of cottage cheese, are excellent sources of calcium and belong in everyone's diet throughout life. Shoot for two or even three servings a day. Don't like milk? Enjoy some yogurt. Or cheese. Even ice cream. Just be sure to choose the nonfat or low-fat varieties. Read the nutrition information labels on dairy foods and you'll see how easy it is to boost your intake of that mineral.

Some dietitians recommend canned salmon as a calcium source, but this assumes that you'll mix the bones in with the fish as you make, say, a salmon salad sandwich. Most people, however, toss the bones away. As for another frequent recommendation to eat a lot of green, leafy vegetables for their calcium content, bear two things in mind. First, few of us are likely to consume enough of those greens each and every day. Second, the calcium in greens is not as well absorbed as that in dairy foods.

All that said, the fact remains that the vast majority of adults will have to use supplements to get the 1,200 to 1,600 mg that women require for both bone health and blood pressure control and the 800 mg that men need. There's another benefit from taking calcium supplements: they appear to lessen the risk of colorectal cancer by limiting rapid cellular growth in that area of the digestive tract.

What sort of calcium supplements should you choose? For bone health, find one that includes vitamin D, which is needed to build bone tissue. Many antacid products are made with calcium carbonate and they add to the day's calcium intake.

Calcium carbonate is the least expensive source of calcium in supplements. Regardless of the form—carbonate, citrate, or gluconate—read the label to determine how much of the actual mineral each tablet provides. Happily, some manufacturers are now offering calcium/magnesium supplements, which I highly recommend.

Magnesium and Blood Pressure

This mineral is the fourth electrolyte needed by the body. As with all the other electrolytes except sodium, we consume less than we should. Most nutritionists do not consider magnesium deficiency to be a major problem, since it's widely available in the food supply and many men and women get an additional amount by way of a multivitamin/mineral supplement. But that doesn't mean we get enough.

Magnesium aids in energy metabolism, promotes proper nerve function, and is involved with muscle activity. It also activates certain enzymes, stabilizes cell structures, and is used for the body to make cell protein, fats, and carbohydrates. Frequently, magnesium supplements are recommended for muscle cramping and other ailments, but our main interest right now is in how this electrolyte can affect blood pressure.

Again, there's a lot of science to back up the notion that we all need to increase our magnesium intake. There have been quite a number of observations that certain countries' populations with higher magnesium consumption through the foods they eat have a reduced risk of developing hypertension. Yet until fairly recently there haven't been the kinds of clinical studies that medical authorities need to make specific recommendations. Here are just three representative studies of that type of scientific investigation.

At Johns Hopkins University in Baltimore, doctors collected data from twenty trials that looked at the effects of magnesium supplementation on blood pressure. They pooled the data to form one "megastudy," in what is termed a *meta-analysis*. In six of the studies, subjects had normal blood pressure; in the others, patients were hypertensive. The data came from 1,220 men and women, and the daily dose of magnesium ranged from 10 to 40 mmol (180 to 720 mg).

Their conclusions are encouraging. For each 10 mmol (180 mg) increase in daily magnesium intake, systolic and diastolic blood pressure decreased by 4.3 and 2.3 mm Hg, respectively. Reductions in blood pressure were dose dependent. That is to say, the more magnesium consumed, the greater the blood pressure decline.

What about the impact of magnesium on the development of heart disease risk? Doctors at the University of Virginia Health System looked at the daily dietary magnesium intake in 7,172 men whose consumption ranged from 50.3 to 1,138 mg (2.8 to 63.2 mmol), with an average of 268 mg (14.9 mmol). During thirty years of follow-up, there were 1,431 cases of coronary heart disease (CHD), and within fifteen years of dietary assessment the age-adjusted incidence of CHD fell significantly in people who had the highest daily magnesium intake (340 mg or more) compared to the lowest (186 mg or less).

In a third study, published in 2004, low levels of magnesium in the blood were associated with an increased risk of stroke. Those low magnesium levels apparently trigger constriction of arteries and increase injury to the endothelium, the lining of arteries. This promotes the development and the progression of heart disease. People with the highest blood concentrations of magnesium had one-third the risk of individuals with the lowest levels.

U.S. nutrition authorities recommend 420 mg (23.3 mmol) for adult men and 320 mg (17.7 mmol) for women as a minimum. Obviously, as we can see in the previous studies, more is better. Shooting for 700 mg (about 40 mmol) is not beyond reason.

A major study tracked 4,637 men and women ages eighteen to thirty for fifteen years. People in the top fourth in terms of magnesium consumption from foods and supplements were less likely to develop high blood pressure, as well as other components of the metabolic syndrome that includes high triglycerides and insulin resistance, a precursor to diabetes.

Where do we get magnesium in the diet? A bit more than 20 percent comes from dairy foods and another 15 percent from meat. That's interesting, since those foods aren't particularly rich in magnesium, but Americans eat a lot of them. Better choices for people desiring to boost their magnesium intake would be a variety of plant foods such as beans, bananas, almonds and cashews, and greens. Clams, by the way, are packed with magnesium; five small ones provide a whopping 112 mg (8.4 mmol).

I think everyone looking to keep his or her blood pressure down should seriously consider magnesium supplements. Daily supplementation of at least 300 mg (16.6 mmol) seems reasonable. That's what I personally take. My supplement contains 300 mg of calcium and 150 mg of magnesium per tablet, and I take two daily.

The Electrolyte Balance

In summary, salt and sodium restriction is difficult to achieve and, when viewed alone, not terribly effective in lowering blood pressure. Few individuals are willing to eat a very bland ultra-low-salt diet for the rest of their lives, and small cutbacks, while advisable, won't do much good if that's all one does.

The answer, I believe and many people agree, is to seek an electrolyte balance of sodium, potassium, calcium, and magnesium. This appears to be the winning formula for blood pressure control.

10

Drink, but Not Too Much

In the past, physicians automatically instructed patients with high blood pressure to stop drinking alcoholic beverages. I clearly remember when my own cardiologist, who had hypertension, was told by his cardiologist, "No more booze." I also remember thinking that I'd have a tougher time giving up my cocktail before dinner or wine with dinner than cutting way back on fat, as I was doing to control my elevated cholesterol.

Happily, today physicians around the world recognize the potential benefits of alcohol consumption, even for people with blood pressure problems. Moderate drinking may actually be good for them. The watchword, of course, is moderation, as it should be for everyone.

More Than a French Paradox

The benefits of alcohol consumption first got public attention when it was noted that the French, who had a very low incidence of heart disease, regularly consumed wine, particularly red wine, with their meals. The French drink a lot of wine, more than they should, and at the time, it wasn't noted that France also has one of the world's highest rates of cirrhosis of the liver.

Since the time of those first reports, researchers around the world have contributed to the now massive body of knowledge regarding the health benefits of alcohol. Looking at mortality rates, it became obvious early on that people who enjoyed a drink or two daily had a lower incidence of cardiovascular disease and lived longer than those who did not drink.

Critics of that observation suggested that investigations included people who had quit drinking owing to illnesses, and that those illnesses, were, in fact responsible for earlier deaths. But when research efforts were refined to exclude such men and women, and focused only on people who had never consumed alcohol, the protection of alcohol held up.

Then it became a question, almost a noisy argument, about what kind of alcohol was best. Was it the red wine favored by the French? Of course, wine merchants touted that. Or was it the beer enjoyed by Germans and others? And what about the spirits preferred by people sipping martinis?

First, let's dispel the superiority of wine in general and red wine in particular. According to Greek researchers in 2005, drinking red wine reduced arterial stiffness in the heart disease patients in their study. As Dr. Emmanouil Karatzis of Athens said, "This is very important considering the fact that patients' vessels are already stiff and this is a major cause of increased blood pressure and consequently increased risk for cardiovascular events." Yet these benefits were also enjoyed by people who drank dealcoholized red wine.

This added one more bit of data to the argument that the benefits of red wine come from the type of antioxidants termed polyphenols and flavonoids. Those chemical substances never get into white wine, since grape skins are removed at the start of the fermentation process. But one can very easily get those polyphenols and flavonoids from red grape juice or pomegranate juice. Or, for that matter, from green tea and a wide variety of fruits and vegetables. Or from beer.

My wife enjoys a cosmopolitan martini now and then, and I make it for her with a splash of pomegranate juice. That brings me back to the issue of which alcoholic beverage is best for heart protection. The short, simple answer is that all kinds of drinks provide benefits equally. It turns out that the alcohol itself yields good things for the body.

More about that in a moment. First, though, what about all those studies showing that men and women who drink wine regularly, rather than either beer or spirits, have a significantly lower rate of heart disease and suffer fewer heart attacks and strokes? It turns out that it's more about the lifestyles of wine lovers than about the wine itself.

Quite a few papers in the medical literature have actually made that point. One of the most recent came from Danish investigators in 2006. Wine drinkers in the Copenhagen study have healthier diets than do people who prefer beer. They buy and eat more fruits, vegetables, olives, low-fat cheese, and cooking oil. Beer drinkers in Denmark, on the other hand, consume fast food, soft drinks, sugar, and saturated and trans fats. To add insult to injury, those wine drinkers were better educated, healthier, and leaner. California investigators have come to the same conclusion about wine drinkers in that state. And, it appears, the same applies to French wine drinkers.

The Benefits of Alcohol

Alcohol, whatever your preference of drink, works its wonders in many ways. The most notable is by raising levels of the protective, "good" HDL cholesterol. This is pretty much a linear phenomenon. The more one drinks, the higher the HDL goes. But, of course, there's the standing caveat of moderation, which I'll define shortly.

Recent investigations have also revealed that alcohol reduces inflammation in the arteries. Doctors have noted that people with heart disease have higher levels of inflammation and, conversely, individuals with little inflammation are at lessened risk of developing the disease and/or suffering a heart attack or a stroke.

There are more than 1,000 English-language papers analyzing the relationship between alcohol usage and the incidence of stroke. Light to moderate alcohol intake has been reported to reduce the rate of all types of stroke, based on a long-term, ongoing study of physicians conducted at Harvard University. Grouped together, studies done from 1966 to 2002 on the link between alcohol and stroke show a decreased risk, and such findings have been reported around the world.

One of the most recent studies comes from Columbia University in New York. There doctors worked with 3,176 mostly Hispanic subjects. The men and women were divided into four groups: those who reported (1) drinking no alcoholic beverages during the past year, (2) moderate consumption of at least one drink per month but no more than two drinks daily, (3) intermediate intake of more than two but fewer than five drinks a day, or (4) heavy drinking of at least five alcoholic beverages daily. During the years of follow-up, moderate drinkers had a 33 percent lower risk of stroke compared with people who were nondrinkers during the previous year.

Alcohol also improves insulin resistance, a component of the so-called metabolic syndrome that predisposes men and women to diabetes and increases the risk of having a heart attack or a stroke. It improves the ability of arteries to dilate to allow for greater blood flow when needed. Alcohol also reduces the risk of developing blood clots by cutting down levels of fibrinogen, a component in the clotting process.

What about hypertensive patients specifically? While most studies in the medical literature have been done with patients who have a variety of levels of blood pressure, rather than focusing on hypertensive individuals, it appears that alcohol's benefits extend to the latter as well. A 2004 study, for example, showed that light to moderate alcohol intake appears to be associated with reduced cardiovascular disease mortality, from both heart attacks and strokes. That research was also conducted with physicians in the Harvard University study.

How Much Should You Drink and How Often?

A lot of people use the word *moderate* without giving much thought to a precise meaning or definition. When it comes to alcohol consumption, medical authorities are virtually unanimous in their recommendations. Moderate means no more than one drink daily for women and two drinks a day for men. One drink is defined as 12 ounces of beer (less for brews that are higher than usual in alcohol content), 5 ounces of wine with an average of 12 percent alcohol, or 1.5 ounces of 80-proof distilled spirits such as scotch whisky, gin, vodka, or bourbon.

Consumption frequency also comes into play. Based on a giant collection of data from 32,826 women and 18,225 men, Harvard researchers concluded that drinking at least three to four days a week is associated with a lowered risk of heart attack. The lowest risk was seen in people drinking three to seven days a week. Another investigation revealed that drinking three to six alcoholic beverages weekly lowers the tendency of blood to clot, but that there was no additional benefit beyond six weekly drinks.

Truth be told, however, heavier alcohol consumption provides other protective benefits against heart disease. Almost grudgingly, a 2005 commentary in the British medical journal *The Lancet* pointed out that during autopsies, the coronary arteries of alcoholics are frequently relatively "clean," indicating a linear level of protection, whether from elevated HDL cholesterol, reduced levels of inflammation, or whatever.

But the authors of that commentary, from the University of Auckland in New Zealand, also note the significant negative effects of heavy alcohol usage. Once again, medical authorities are unanimous in strongly advocating against heavy drinking, describing the benefits and the ill effects of alcohol consumption as a "J-shaped" curve.

As men and women go from being nondrinkers, in studies corroborated again and again all over the globe, to light or moderate drinkers, their risk of cardiovascular disease decreases. But as study populations in general, and individuals in particular, graduate from moderate to heavy drinking, the risk of all-cause mortality goes up. Canadian research has shown that women in particular appear to be more at risk of developing hypertension when alcohol consumption goes beyond moderate levels. In that 2006 investigation, doctors found that heavy alcohol use raised blood pressure levels throughout both the day and the night.

The heavier the drinking, the greater the risk. Alcoholism increases in heavy drinkers as do accidental injuries and deaths, especially on the highways. Cirrhosis of the liver becomes more likely. The heart muscle, protected by light to moderate drinking, becomes damaged by heavy intake. Binge drinking, defined as five or more drinks a day, poses particular ill effects.

Alcohol and Blood Pressure

A 2006 report issued by the American Heart Association points to clinical trials showing that consuming less alcohol reduces both systolic and diastolic blood pressure. However, the AHA says, evidence supports the fact that moderate alcohol intake is effective in lowering blood pressure. The group concludes that alcohol consumption should be limited to no more than two drinks a day for men and one for women.

There has been considerable discussion in the world's medical literature and at medical conferences as to whether physicians should actually advocate initiation of alcohol consumption for patients who currently do not drink. Certainly, there is unequivocal proof of the cardiovascular benefits, but there is also unequivocal proof of the potential downside of drinking, both for the individual and for society as a whole. The horrors of deaths to drunk drivers and their victims come vividly and dramatically to mind, as does the sociological impact of alcoholism on the individual and his or her family.

Doctors conclude, and I strongly agree, that if you currently enjoy light to moderate alcohol consumption, continue to do so. But if you are a nondrinker, do not begin to drink just to protect your heart. Whether you lift a glass of an alcoholic or a nonalcoholic beverage, I end this chapter with a toast: "To good health and happiness!"

11

Lower Your Cholesterol, Lower Your Blood Pressure

What is a chapter on cholesterol doing in a book on blood pressure? For openers, elevated cholesterol levels in the blood represent one of the Big Three risk factors for cardiovascular disease, along with high blood pressure and cigarette smoking. But there's even more reason to include this chapter. It now appears that blood pressure and cholesterol are more closely related than anyone previously thought.

In 2005, research demonstrated that lowering blood pressure brings cholesterol counts down at the same time. That next year, doctors examining data from an ongoing study of thousands of women found that high cholesterol levels predict future hypertension. The higher a woman's cholesterol during middle age, the more likely she'll later develop high blood pressure. Women in this particular subset of the investigation were at least forty-five years of age in 1992, and none had either high cholesterol or elevated blood pressure. After nearly eleven years, 4,593 women, nearly one-third, had developed high blood pressure. Those with the highest total/HDL ratios had a 34 percent greater likelihood of getting hypertension. Conversely, women with high HDL counts had a 16 percent lower than average risk. And, also in 2006, that link was extended to men by way of the Physicians' Health Study, a similar ongoing investigation of thousands of men whose diets, lifestyle habits, and development and progression of disease are carefully tracked.

In this particular case, the study period was just over fourteen years. During that time, 1,019 male physicians in a group of 3,110 developed hypertension. Harvard researchers then compared the cholesterol levels of those men with the cholesterol levels of people whose blood pressure remained in the normal range. Individuals having the highest levels of total cholesterol were 23 percent more likely to develop hypertension than were men with the lowest counts. And men with the highest ratio of total cholesterol to the protective "good" HDL cholesterol had a 54 percent greater risk of developing high blood pressure.

The message is simple. You kill two birds with one stone by getting your cholesterol under control whether you're a man or a woman. Reduce the risk posed by that factor and you'll also cut the chances of developing hypertension later in life.

Having personally fought high cholesterol levels since 1984 at the time of my second coronary bypass surgery and having written extensively on cholesterol, I think I'm in a good position to give you some sound advice. Back in 1984, my total cholesterol was a dangerously high 269. By following the program I developed, I got it down to 184 in just eight weeks. In 1987, I shared my regimen with the world in the book *The 8-Week Cholesterol Cure* and in the 2002 complete rewrite and update, *The New 8-Week Cholesterol Cure*.

Obviously, I can't cover all the details I discuss in those two books, but I think I can give you enough information in this chapter to get you solidly on the road to cholesterol control. The bottom-line promise, as has been true since 1987, is that you can get your cholesterol down to safe levels in just eight weeks. The program I'm going to outline has worked for millions of men and women and can work for you.

What Is Cholesterol?

That's still the first question most people ask. Simply stated, cholesterol is a chemical substance that is essential for bodily functions, including digestion, manufacture of hormones, formation of cell walls, and protection of nerve endings. We can't live without it. It's in practically every tissue of our bodies.

That's the good news. The bad news is that when there's too much cholesterol, it tends to cause blockage in our arteries, leading to heart disease, heart attacks, and strokes. Cholesterol has also been linked with Alzheimer's disease.

The substance itself isn't soluble in water or, on a more practical level, in the bloodstream. So cholesterol is transported through the body in a variety of envelopes made of fat and protein called lipoproteins. Cholesterol transported in a low-density lipoprotein envelope tends to be deposited in damaged regions of our arteries. That's a bad thing, so we call LDL (low-density lipoprotein) cholesterol "bad." But in the body's system of balances, we also have cholesterol transported out of those arteries and removed from the bloodstream by HDL (high-density lipoprotein). We call that combination the "good" cholesterol.

Most of the cholesterol in our bloodstream, about 80 percent of it, is made by the body itself, principally in the liver. In an ideal situation, there would be proper balance of the LDL and HDL cholesterol, not too much of the LDL and enough HDL. But nearly 50 percent of men and women inherit a family gene that results in the production of too much LDL and too little HDL. Even with a heart-healthy lifestyle of diet and exercise, such people will still have a cholesterol level that will predispose them to the development of cardiovascular disease and eventual heart attacks and strokes.

The other fatty substances floating around in our blood are the triglycerides. These fats are used by the body for energy and come from the foods we eat. Here, too, some of us just naturally have too much, and our lifestyles boost levels even more, resulting in a risk factor independent of cholesterol.

Wouldn't it be terrific if we could simply tell our livers not to make so much of the bad LDL cholesterol and to make more of the good HDL cholesterol instead? It would be even better if we could cut down the amount of triglycerides in our blood as well. The good news is that we can do just that, without having to resort to prescription drugs.

Have Your Cholesterol Level Tested

You have no idea whether you have a high cholesterol level or not without testing for it in the blood. Perversely, there are no symptoms of its elevation, and someone who is obese and sedentary may have a low level while a lean, athletic person's cholesterol might be dangerously high. Not fair, is it?

Fortunately, cholesterol testing is quite simple and provides vital information for us to fight against heart disease. Simply schedule a day and a time to visit your doctor's office, preferably in the morning before you've eaten anything that day. You'll want to get what physicians call a "lipid panel," which consists of measurement of total cholesterol (TC), LDL cholesterol, HDL cholesterol, ratio of total to good cholesterol, and triglycerides (TG). Request a measurement of your glucose levels as well; they should be less than 126, ideally just under 100. You can get those tests done at the same time you have your blood pressure measured. You should have the results in just a few days.

In the United States, we use mg/dl (milligrams per deciliter) in measurements of total, LDL, and HDL cholesterol and for glucose and triglycerides. Virtually all other countries use mmol/L (millimoles per liter), and some U.S. laboratories are now using that international designation in test reports. Here are the equations to convert from mg/dl to mmol/L. Using a calculator makes the effort a lot easier.

> For cholesterol (total, LDL, and HDL), multiply mg/dl by 0.02586 to get mmol/L.
> To go from mmol/L to mg/dl, multiply by 38.7.
> For triglycerides, multiply mg/dl by 0.01129 to get mmol/L.
> To go from mmol/L to mg//dl, multiply by 88.6.
> For glucose, multiply mg/dl by 0.055 to get mmol/L.
> To go from mmol/L to mg/dl, multiply by 18.0.

Medical authorities state that TC should be no more than 200 (measured as milligrams per deciliter) or 4.1 millimoles per liter. That's fine, I suppose, if there's no family history of heart disease and if you have no other risk factors going on at the same time, such as elevated blood pressure, sedentary behavior, smoking, diabetes, and overweight. But the fact is that the lower you can get your TC, the better. Risk begins to increase well before the previously mentioned cut-offs.

Levels of LDL should be lower than 100 mg/dl. Again, the lower the better. Conversely, we want HDL to be as high as possible, with women's levels no lower than 45 and men's no lower than 40. The ratio of TC/HDL has been shown to be an even more accurate predictor of risk than is TC or LDL alone. We want your ratio to be no more than 4.5 for men and 4.0 for women. Finally, TG counts should be under 150, and ideally down to about 100 or so.

I strongly suggest that you ask your doctor's office to send a printed copy of your report so you can keep it in a file and use it for comparison in the years to come. Don't accept a statement that "Everything's okay." Learn what your actual numbers are. Each of us should maintain a personal health file in our homes. Put your cholesterol report in that file, along with your blood pressure measurement and other medical information. (When did you last have a booster shot for tetanus, for example?)

Okay, you've had your test and you see that your numbers need improvement. No problem. Controlling cholesterol levels—all your lipids—is far easier today than it was back in 1984 when I began my own efforts. Let's start with a cholesterol-lowering diet.

Eat a Heart-Healthy Diet

Essentially, the diet that's ideal for controlling blood pressure, as described in chapter 12, is just what you need for cholesterol lowering and maintenance as well. So here I'll just discuss a few of the principal points that particularly pertain to cholesterol.

It turns out that not all fats and oils are the villains the medical community thought them to be in the 1980s. Recommendations then were to reduce all fats. Today we've refined this advice, knowing that it's only the saturated and the trans fats and oils we need to limit.

Saturated fats are found in meats, dairy foods, and palm kernel and coconut oils. But that doesn't mean we have to become vegetarians. Simply opt for lean cuts of beef, lamb, and pork and nonfat or at least low-fat dairy products. Read food package labels to avoid palm kernel and coconut oils.

A recent study in the *American Journal of Clinical Nutrition* showed that replacing some of the carbohydrates in the diet with lean red meat actually lowered blood pressure. The replaced carbs included white bread, pasta, white rice, and cakes and cookies. Ultimately, it's a question of balance, but this study shows that there's no need to exclude lean cuts of red meat from a heart-smart diet.

The last thing you'd want to do is eliminate dairy foods in a misguided effort to avoid saturated fat or to lower calorie intake. We all need calcium for good bone health and for a variety of body functions. Moreover, it appears that people who consume the most low-fat dairy foods have half the incidence of hypertension, according to Spanish investigators who looked at the diets of nearly 6,000 well-educated men and women who had normal blood pressure at the beginning of the study and who developed hypertension over a twenty-seven-month study.

My first thought in reading the article was that it must be the calcium in dairy, but that, it turned out, was not the case at all, even though calcium itself is indeed part of the electrolyte balance needed to control blood pressure. In this study, however, people getting as much calcium from other sources did not enjoy the same protection. Nor did individuals who consumed whole-fat dairy foods. Only the low-fat dairy products provided blood pressure maintenance.

Trans fats are found in manufactured and processed foods such as crackers, cookies, and other baked goods; in deep-fried fast foods; and in nondairy creamers, dessert toppings, and so on. When shopping, look for "partially hydrogenated" oils in the ingredients list. The process of hydrogenation, done to lengthen shelf life and to improve taste, produces the trans-fatty acids that not only raise LDL but also lower HDL. They even contribute to inflammation in the arteries, another risk factor for heart disease. As of January 1, 2006, all packaged foods sold in the United States must include listings of the amount of trans fat along with saturated fat on the

Nutrition Facts label. Note, however, that because of the way the law is worded, certain food items such as nondairy creamers are allowed to say on their front label "0 g trans fats" if the amount of trans fats is less than 1 gram per serving. If the manufacturer states that one serving equals one teaspoon, despite the fact that many people use much more than that in a cup of coffee, then legally the manufacturer has complied with the FDA's ruling. The wise consumer needs to also read the ingredients list where "partially hydrogenated vegetable oil" is listed as a primary ingredient. Trans-fatty acids also occur in the oils used in fast-food restaurants for deep-frying, especially when the oil is repeatedly heated.

That's it. That's all you need to watch for in the way of fats. We've learned that virtually all other fats are either good for your heart or are neutral in their effects. That's particularly true for the omega-3 fatty acids found in fish. While we want to choose lean cuts of beef, opt for the fattiest fish, including salmon, herring, and sardines. The omega-3 fatty acids protect the heart by limiting the formation of blood clots, reducing arterial inflammation, and lowering both triglycerides and blood pressure.

Until the 1990s, we thought it was best to cut way back on nuts of all sorts, as they are quite high in fat. But research has now documented that nuts are actually good for your heart. In fact, people who snack on nuts regularly, even daily, are more protected against heart disease than people who don't eat nuts. Nuts of all kinds— almonds, walnuts, pecans, cashews, peanuts, and peanut butter— have little saturated fat. Instead they are rich in polyunsaturated fat that improves cholesterol levels.

When shopping for margarine, look for soft types sold in tubs rather than in sticks. But read the labels to choose the brands that are lowest in saturated and trans fats.

I personally use and enjoy a wide variety of oils. Olive oil is great for sautéing certain foods and is a staple in the Mediterranean diet that's best for blood pressure control. Canola oil is similarly rich in the monounsaturated fatty acids that lower cholesterol when they're used to replace saturated fats. Canola oil is best when you're cooking at higher temperatures or when you don't want the oil to add a distinctive flavor. Of all the oils in my pantry, I use canola oil most frequently, virtually on a daily basis. I like walnut oil for salads, mixed with raspberry vinegar as a dressing. Peanut oil gives Asian foods a wonderful taste. Other oils, including soybean, safflower, and corn oils, are low in saturated fats and high in poly-unsaturated fatty acids.

Although all healthy diets should include a spectrum of fruits and vegetables—at the very least, five servings daily—and whole-grain breads and cereals, cutting too far back on animal protein and healthful fats and oils can tip the scales in the wrong direction. A very-low-fat diet that's also low in protein is not only boring and not very tasty but also tends to raise levels of triglycerides and to lower the protective HDL. Again, go for lean cuts of meats and poultry, lots of fish and seafood, nonfat or low-fat dairy foods, and oils such as olive and canola—limited only by calories if you eat too much.

Numerous studies have determined that a diet low in saturated and trans fats can typically reduce cholesterol levels from 5 to 8 per-cent. That's a good start, of course, but many men and women will need to do more. As noted, however, cutting too far back on fat and protein and eating a diet heavily dominated by plant-based foods may lower the total and the LDL cholesterol, but HDL and triglyc-erides will be adversely affected. Remember that the ratio of total to HDL cholesterol is a better predictor of heart disease risk than either total or LDL cholesterol.

You can improve that ratio by including foods in your diet that are rich in soluble fiber. Foods such as oatmeal and oat bran, dried beans of all sorts (pintos, garbanzos, kidney beans, and so on), figs, and barley are all great sources of that specialized fiber. Regularly including them in your diet can bring your LDL cholesterol down by another 5 percent or more while not lowering your HDL choles-terol at all. As a special bonus, research has shown that a diet rich in soluble fiber also promotes lower blood pressure.

There are two soluble fiber supplements that lower choles-terol. Metamucil (psyllium) has been shown to be quite effective, but many people dislike the gritty, thick consistency when it's mixed with water or other fluids. My personal choice is Profibe, developed by a physician at the University of Florida. Profibe is made from citrus fiber—pectin—and one scoop supplies 6 grams of soluble fiber. I routinely add a scoop to all my smoothies, and it can be added to orange juice, water, or any beverage without becoming thick like psyllium. You can get more information and place orders at www.profibe.com. It is not sold in stores at this time.

Blocking Cholesterol from the Foods You Eat

Let's say that you're right on the border between a healthy and a dangerous cholesterol level. A 10 percent reduction might be all you need. Well, nature has provided a great solution by way of the plant world's equivalent of cholesterol itself.

Just as all animal tissues and foods contain cholesterol, which is needed for life itself, all plants have phytosterols, plant sterols. The molecular structures of cholesterol and phytosterols are virtually identical (see the illustration). Because they are so similar, the human body cannot tell the difference.

As such, phytosterols are readily accepted into the receptor sites, specialized cells called micelles, that transport cholesterol directly into the bloodstream from the digestive tract. Those micelles are located in the first third of the small intestine. Early research showed that only a limited amount of cholesterol could be transported into the blood from the gastrointestinal (GI) tract at a time.

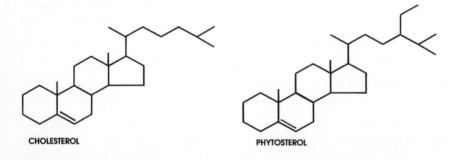

CHOLESTEROL   PHYTOSTEROL

Give those receptor sites phytosterols and the sites accept them as if they were cholesterol, thus blocking cholesterol itself. The trick, then, is to take concentrated phytosterols in tablet form at the beginning of a meal, especially meals containing animal foods that have cholesterol. Bear in mind that all animal foods have essentially the same amount of cholesterol whether they're lean or fatty; in fact, chicken breast has more cholesterol than beef does.

Some foods, of course, have more cholesterol than others. Eggs, organ meats, and shrimp are particularly cholesterol-rich. For about ten years, I never ate a single egg yolk. Since discovering how well the phytosterols work, I now regularly enjoy eggs in all forms and my cholesterol tests have never been better. I just swallow a couple of tablets at the start of the meal.

So, one mode of action for the phytosterols is to inhibit or completely block absorption of dietary cholesterol into the bloodstream. But they work in another, entirely different, way as well. That's by preventing the recycling of bile, made from cholesterol, following a meal. Phytosterols attach to the bile, which is then eliminated in the bowel movement. That's why taking the plant sterols improves cholesterol levels even when they're used before meals that have little or no cholesterol at all.

Between those two modes of action, including phytosterols on a regular, daily basis will lower your total cholesterol by about 10 percent and your LDL by up to 14 percent, while not reducing your HDL at all. The result is a much improved ratio and a decreased risk of developing or worsening heart disease.

Sound too good to be true? More than twelve hundred research studies, conducted at top medical centers around the world and published in the most prestigious medical journals, document both the safety and efficacy of phytosterols in cholesterol control. They are completely safe not only because they are naturally found in plants but also because they never enter the bloodstream. After blocking the receptor micelles for probably one to two hours, they are rejected, owing to the slight difference in molecular structure, and are eliminated by the body. Even children and pregnant women can take them without fear.

Phytosterol supplement tablets are widely available, but I am aware of only one brand formulated for immediate release. Why is that important? Most tablets take twenty to thirty minutes to dissolve in the stomach before they can release their plant sterols to block cholesterol. Therefore, you must either swallow the tablets ahead of time or accept the fact that cholesterol will compete with the phytosterol at the receptor sites in the digestive tract. Some of the cholesterol will get into the bloodstream. If the phytosterol is immediately released, though, it goes straight to those receptor micelles and leaves no room for cholesterol so that you don't need to time the dosage and you'll get more improvement in your cholesterol.

The immediate-release formulation of phytosterols is made by Endurance Products Company, based outside of Portland, Oregon. Its Web site is www.endur.com. This is the same company that makes the best formulation of my favorite method of cholesterol control, niacin. Place orders outside the United States at www .endur.com; click on Customer Service page, International Orders. Take two 450 mg tablets at the start of two major meals daily to block the absorption of cholesterol in the foods you eat, inhibit the recycling of bile made of cholesterol, and achieve a cholesterol reduction in your bloodstream of up to 10 percent.

A variety of foods are now fortified with the heart-healthy plant sterols. Look for products bearing the names Corowise and Heart-Wise, such as Minute Maid HeartWise orange juice and Health Valley HeartWise cereals. For more information visit www.corowise.com.

Niacin: Your Heart's Best Friend

Niacin is a vitamin, B3, but when taken in doses larger than needed for nutrition, it is the best agent in the world for cholesterol control. Not even prescription drugs come close. That's because niacin affects the entire spectrum in the lipid panel.

Niacin supplementation causes total and LDL cholesterol levels to fall by an average of 20 to 40 percent. This fall has been documented again and again at major medical centers worldwide. Protective levels of the good HDL cholesterol rise. Improvements in HDL occur in patients with both elevated and normal triglycerides, whereas the drug gemfibrozil, for example, works only when triglycerides are up. Often HDL improvements can be made even with niacin doses as low as 500 mg, as documented by physicians in Israel and elsewhere. At the Mayo Clinic in Rochester, Minnesota, sixty-three participants in a cardiac rehabilitation program who had low HDL levels experienced an average 18 percent increase with niacin. Doctors at the Ochsner Clinic in New Orleans achieved a 32 percent HDL improvement.

Triglyceride measurements fall precipitously with niacin. The higher the initial levels, the greater the response. In a study supported by the National Institutes of Health in the United States, triglycerides fell an average of 52 percent. Other studies show 15 to 30 percent reductions or higher, depending on the dosage.

Only niacin offers benefits in regard to newly determined, independent risk factors for the development and progression of heart disease and the incidence of heart attacks and strokes. It lowers levels of a particularly nasty variant of LDL termed *lipoprotein(a)*. The vitamin improves the balance of the hormonelike substances called prostaglandins, with the detrimental thromboxane falling and the protective prostacycline going up. Activity of blood platelets, cells involved in the clotting process, decrease, resulting in fewer clots that can lead to heart attacks.

Doctors now recognize that small, dense particles of LDL cholesterol are more dangerous than larger, buoyant particles. Niacin causes a shift from small, dense LDL to large, buoyant particles. No prescription drug can do that!

Finally, niacin lowers levels of inflammation in the arteries. As total and LDL cholesterol fall along with lipoprotein(a), HDL goes up, other benefits occur, and the measurements of inflammation decrease.

Niacin can be used either alone, which, for most men and women seeking cholesterol control, is enough, or in combination with the statin drugs. In fact, research at the University of Washington and elsewhere proves that the combination represents the state-of-the-art approach to aggressive cholesterol control, completely stopping the progression of heart disease and even reversing blockage of the arteries.

In view of the current medical consensus that LDL cholesterol levels should be as low as possible, especially for people with a personal or family history of heart disease, and that all aspects of the lipid profile should be controlled as well, niacin is essential. One could also make a strong case for saying that a person at risk of having a heart attack or a stroke is not being effectively treated if he or she is not taking niacin as part of the total heart-healthy regimen.

Niacin benefits heart health when used at dosages significantly higher than when the vitamin is viewed in nutritional terms. It works its wonders in the liver, the principal site of cholesterol manufacture by the body. As such, niacin usage should be monitored by your physician. Regular tests will determine not only your cholesterol levels but also the health of your liver. Be sure to discuss this with your doctor. He or she will certainly be aware of just how well niacin works as your heart's best friend. If not, point your doctor to the references cited at the end of this book.

Historically, the biggest problem with niacin was the virtual certainty of flushing of the skin. This has been likened to the hot flashes experienced by women going through menopause. My comparison is to rolling around in the sand after getting a nasty sunburn. Not very pleasant. But that's history, because there are now sustained-release formulations of niacin that practically eliminate flushing by gradually allowing niacin to enter the bloodstream. The best of these is made by the Endurance Products Company. Its product, Endur-acin, has been extensively clinically tested and evaluated at the University of Minnesota and elsewhere for both safety and efficacy. It is recommended by doctors throughout the United States, including Dr. Thomas Pickering, a highly recognized authority on blood pressure control and hypertension at the Cornell Medical Center in New York. Look for it at www.endur.com. Your heart will thank you for it! You can e-mail orders outside the United States at www.endur.com; click on Customer Service page, International Orders. In your e-mail, indicate that you would like to purchase Endur-acin to be shipped. The company will e-mail you back with specific prices and procedures. Unfortunately, they do not accept credit cards, and you will have to send a check in advance.

The dosage determined to be the safest and most effective is one 500 mg tablet of Endur-acin three times daily for a total of 1,500 mg a day. That's much lower than was previously used in medical research with inferior formulations of niacin. Most individuals take it with meals, as a way to remember to take all three tablets daily, but the scheduling is not absolutely important. For example, I take my evening dosage at bedtime, when I brush my teeth. What matters is to remember to take it three times a day. To help me remember, I keep some in my car, office, kitchen, attaché and travel cases, and golf bag. I know how important niacin is to my heart health—I really believe it's the single most vital thing I did to save my own life—and I don't want to forget to take even one dose. But if you do happen to forget, say, the midday tablet, double up the dosage in the evening.

A prescription-only sustained-release niacin, NiaSpan, has been widely promoted to doctors, but the formulation, frankly, is inferior to that of Endur-acin. Readers of mine whose doctors convinced them to switch from Endur-acin to NiaSpan have written to me complaining of flushing and gastric disturbances.

I want you to know that I don't own stock in the Endurance Products Company and that I don't get a cent for recommending Endur-acin. I do so because I believe it is the best niacin formulation in the world, and I want my readers to have the best.

Speaking of the best, please be sure to avoid the worst! There are unscrupulous companies that sell products labeled as "No-Flush Niacin." These are either niacinamide, a metabolite of niacin, or inositol hexanicotinate. Neither of these has any effect whatsoever on cholesterol levels. Despite claims to the contrary, neither has been shown to affect cholesterol at all. Niacin breaks down to niacinamide in the body, but only the niacin, not the amide form, has any benefit. And the inositol hexanicotinate, simply enough, does not provide any niacin at all, as proved in clinical studies. Please do not believe any Internet advertisements or claims made by salespeople in health food stores or elsewhere.

Bear in mind that niacin works to lower cholesterol levels and produce its other benefits at much higher doses than in the amount that's needed as a nutrient. In that regard, it is working like a drug in the liver to limit LDL and raise HDL production. Talk with your doctor about niacin in your own case to find out if there are reasons you shouldn't take it, such as existing liver problems. When you take niacin, your doctor will want to check your liver enzymes periodically to make sure your body is handling it without any problems.

I've taken niacin since 1984, and Endur-acin in particular since 1988, without any difficulties whatever. I truly believe it has played a major role in saving my life.

Additional Options for Cholesterol Control

For most men and women, a heart-healthy diet that's rich in soluble fiber and supplemented with phytosterols and niacin will control cholesterol very nicely. In fact, you can expect that your doctor will be amazed at your results. But there are other natural approaches as well.

Red yeast rice has been a staple in Chinese medicine and cooking for centuries. It has been clinically proven to reduce LDL cholesterol. That makes sense, since red yeast rice is a natural source of the statin drug lovastatin, although products made from red yeast rice contain a much lower level of the substance. It's available in pharmacies and health food stores.

Policosanol was first researched by doctors in Cuba. It is derived from the waxy outer coating of sugarcane, which is grown extensively in that country. Studies showed its effectiveness to be equal to that of low doses of prescription statin drugs. Very little research, however, has been done outside of Cuba, and results of that research have never been published in any major medical journal. The death knell for policosanol was sounded with the publication of a report in the May 17, 2006, issue of the *Journal of the American Medical Association*. German researchers did what is termed an elegant study that was conducted at multiple medical centers, was double-blind and placebo controlled, and used exactly the dosage and the form previously claimed to be effective. Even at twice the usual recommended dosage, there was absolutely no benefit, zero cholesterol reduction. Save your money; policosanol does not work.

Prescription Drugs for Lowering Cholesterol

In 1984, when I began my own fight against heart disease in general and cholesterol in particular, there were only two prescription drugs available. These were in the class known as bile-sequestering resins, which worked by binding to bile from the digestive tract and removing it from the body, causing cholesterol to be drawn from the bloodstream to make more.

Both brands of those resin drugs were particularly nasty to take. Imagine pouring foul-tasting and foul-smelling sand into a glass of water or juice, swirling it into a slurry, and gulping it down before it could settle out. Now do that two, three, even four times daily as prescribed. Then settle into the gastric disturbances that were common.

I wanted no part of them and went on to develop the natural alternative program of oat bran and niacin, along with a low-fat diet. (Some people would say that niacin is actually a drug since it works very differently in large doses than it would as a nutrient. And, as stated, niacin calls for medical supervision when taken in large dosages.)

The next class of drugs that came along were the so-called fibrate derivatives, including gemfibrozil (Lopid). They did an adequate job of reducing triglycerides and raising HDL but achieved only marginal LDL improvements. Niacin did a better job on all fronts, although at the time doctors thought that huge doses, up to 8 grams a day, were needed and only the standard crystalline niacin was available. The flushing and the gastric disturbances understandably made patient compliance poor. Endur-acin, of course, ended those problems.

Next we come to the modern class of prescribed cholesterol-lowering drugs, the statins. These are the drugs seen frequently on TV and in magazine advertisements. The first of this class, lovastatin

(Mevacor), got FDA clearance in the United States in August 1987. Along with lovastatin, there are currently six statin drugs on the market; the others are simvastatin (Zocor), pravastatin (Pravacol), fluvastatin (Lescol), atorvastatin (Lipitor), and rosuvastatin (Crestor). A seventh statin, cerivastatin (Baycol), was taken off the market following drug-related deaths.

All of these drugs have the same mode of action. They are HMG co-A reductase inhibitors. Simply stated, they inhibit the liver's production of an enzyme that's essential to the manufacture of cholesterol. These are very powerful drugs, the most potent of which are atorvastatin and rosuvastatin, and are capable of reducing cholesterol, especially LDL, by as much as 50 percent or even more.

In all honesty, the drugs appear to be relatively safe as a class. They have been used for two decades and have been prescribed to many millions of men and women around the world. Studies have demonstrated that they can prevent heart attacks and strokes and save lives by dramatically reducing cholesterol. Obviously, there were terrible problems with cerivastatin (Baycol). And the British medical journal *The Lancet* has asked for a recall of rosuvastatin (Crestor), citing poor research data and potential side effects involving the liver and the kidneys and muscle damage. Consumer advocates in the United States have also called for FDA to reverse its approval.

People taking statin drugs should have regular liver function tests, typically every six months or so. Those tests measure levels of liver enzymes. It's also important to report any muscle aches or weakness when taking these drugs, as they might be early signs of muscle damage that could become severe. Permanent deterioration of muscle tissue, termed rhabdomyolysis, is an infrequent but very real adverse reaction. Many doctors believe that such problems can be avoided by limiting the dosage. If greater cholesterol reduction than that achieved at a low dose is required, combination therapy can bring a patient to goal levels.

Research at the University of California at San Diego indicates that the side effects of the statin drugs may be due to the depletion of a substance naturally produced by the body called coenzyme

Q10, or simply CoQ10. It turns out that the very same enzyme needed to make cholesterol in the liver is necessary for the production of CoQ10.

CoQ10 is found throughout the body, literally in all tissues. Another name for it is ubiquinone, indicating that it is ubiquitous—everywhere—in the body. It is involved in energy production within muscle cells. As we age, CoQ10 production declines. Statin drugs further deplete the body's CoQ10 resources. Based on their preliminary, currently unpublished investigations, the U.C. San Diego researchers suggest that all patients taking statin drugs take supplemental CoQ10 as a safeguard against muscle damage. They recommend from 150 mg to 600 mg daily, depending on the dosage of statin drugs taken.

There are a lot of CoQ10 products on the market. Prices vary and so does quality and effectiveness. The best raw material for CoQ10 is produced through a yeast process by the Japanese company Kanaka. And the best formulation is in an oil base, such as the one made by Healthy Origins. It is the formulation used in the U.C. San Diego study. You can find it in retail stores and at www.healthyorigins.com. That company also makes a number of blood pressure–lowering supplements, my secret weapons against high blood pressure, I write about elsewhere in the book.

Statin drug takers should also be aware of a little known food-drug interaction involving grapefruit. Several studies have all come to the same conclusion. Grapefruit and grapefruit juice vastly increase the amount of a statin drug in the blood—by as much as twelve-fold. Although grapefruit is an excellent food and a great source of vitamin C, statin users should probably avoid it.

While statin drugs can dramatically lower LDL cholesterol, they do very little to raise HDL, to lower triglycerides or lipoprotein(a), or to improve the other parameters, which I explained earlier, that niacin influences beneficially. There's no doubt in my mind that niacin is the better choice.

But some men and women have extremely elevated levels of LDL. For such people, the best approach would be a combination of a low dose of a statin drug and niacin. That would be particularly advisable if the person has already experienced a heart attack or a stroke or has had bypass surgery or an angioplasty. Such individuals need to get their LDL as low as possible, and the best way to achieve that is with the statin/niacin combo. If you're in that position, and your doctor balks at the idea of niacin, ask him or her to look at the medical literature. Otherwise, find another doctor.

Twenty-five years ago, few people knew what cholesterol was or had even heard of it. Today it's a household word. As one of the Big Three risk factors for cardiovascular disease, it's something that just has to be controlled. Doing so is easier and more effective than ever before, and the cholesterol-blood pressure connection has been well established.

12

Eating to Lower
Blood Pressure

During the early 1950s, when I was eight or nine years old, hanging around the kitchen and asking my mother questions about foods and cooking, really getting into it at that early age, a researcher at the University of Minnesota was thinking about food, lifestyle, and health. Dr. Ancel Keys, working with scientists around the world, launched one of the most provocative and influential investigations ever. The Seven Countries Study led the way in our recognizing that how we live and what we eat greatly influences our health. And pestering my mom around the kitchen led me to a lifelong love of food and cooking.

Rates of heart disease were extremely low in Italy, Greece, and Japan, where diets that were low in animal fats and high in fruits, vegetables, seafood, and oils predominated. Where dietary and lifestyle patterns were reversed, in Yugoslavia, Finland, the Netherlands, and the United States, the incidence of heart disease soared. Careful research continued through the 1960s and 1970s. Now, in the twenty-first century, we have pretty much worked out the details as to how to keep our hearts and bodies healthy and prevent cardiovascular disease in general and heart attacks and strokes in particular.

We live in a much smaller world today, in a cultural sense. Crete, a Greek island where those early studies were done, now has

McDonald's and other fast-food restaurants, and the traditional Mediterranean diet is sadly on the wane. Similar changes have occurred in Japan and Italy, as well as in France, another country where healthy eating and active lifestyles dominated in the past. Not surprisingly, people who have traded olive oil for butter, and soups and fresh fish for cheeseburgers, have seen their cholesterol and blood pressure levels rise. The World Health Organization calculates that 600 million men and women in the world now have hypertension and that 3 million die annually from it.

Conversely, when the traditionally healthy food choices from the Mediterranean and Asia replace poor eating habits in the United States and elsewhere in the world, health improves. The good news is that making these changes does not mean living a life of deprivation. Nor does it mean completely eliminating our favorite regional foods that we've grown up with, wherever we happen to live.

Before getting much further into the science behind heart-healthy nutrition and eating patterns that are known to reduce blood pressure, I want to make it perfectly clear that I love food as much as ever, if not even more. I'm definitely not one of the "Food Police" who take all the joy out of eating. To me, food is a gift to be celebrated not just once in a while but every day! What I've learned is to marry the nutritious and the delicious. In the pages to come, I'll make your mouth water as I show you ways to keep both your heart and your taste buds happy.

Scientific Proof of the Benefits of Heart-Healthy Eating

You'd think that it wouldn't take thousands of doctors, scientists, and nutritionists all over the world to figure out how and what to eat to stay healthy. After all, Grandma said, "Eat your fruits and vegetables." Of course, she was absolutely right, but there's more to it than that. Grandma quite likely kept a coffee can filled with bacon grease to use for cooking, as mine did, and my mother as well.

And what about those tales told in every family about Grandpa Joe or Uncle Peter who ate bacon and eggs every morning, hated fruits and vegetables, and demanded meat and potatoes for dinner seven days a week? "They lived into their nineties and never had a problem." Sure. And there certainly are people who smoke cigarettes all their lives without getting lung cancer or emphysema, but they are the exception to what we now know is the rule.

When I began my career as a medical journalist in the 1960s, many physicians smoked cigarettes. That's not true anymore. You have to look long and hard to find a doctor who smokes.

Take a look around you, as my wife, Dawn, and I did one time while on a vacation cruise in Mexico. We saw a lot of fat people and we saw a lot of old people. But we couldn't spot one person who was both old and fat. You don't have to be a scientist to figure out why. Obese people don't live long.

It's more than just living long, though. Quality of life is as or more important than quantity of life. As the old saying goes, when you have your health you have everything. Hard-core research studies have shown us that you can eat your way to good health. You don't really need the details, but here is some proof of the proverbial pudding.

When doctors came to the realization that fat was associated with cholesterol levels, they threw the baby out with the bath water, recommending a diet that was low in all fat, not just the saturated fats in meats, dairy, and the tropical oils. Yes, when men and women followed that diet, levels of their "bad" LDL cholesterol came down—but so did the "good" HDL that protects the heart. And amounts of an independently harmful blood fat, triglycerides, went up. For all their efforts, after giving up a lot of the foods they enjoyed, such people were actually worse off than before.

Today we know that only two fats hurt the heart. In addition to the saturated fats, trans-fatty acids formed by the partial hydrogenation of otherwise healthy oils such as soybean or sunflower are culprits. They're even worse than saturated fats, in that they lower the levels of both LDL and HDL. You find them in processed, packaged foods such as baked goods and margarines and in deep-fried foods in restaurants. All other fats and oils are either flat-out beneficial or at least neutral in their effects on heart-health parameters, but, especially in the case of those nasty trans fats, it took decades for us to learn these lessons through painstaking research projects all over the world.

Researchers from Denmark collaborated with doctors at the University of Wollongong in New South Wales, Australia, to determine the effects of saturated, monounsaturated, and omega-3 fatty acids on blood pressure in healthy subjects. They found that decreasing the saturated fats and increasing the monounsaturated led to decreased blood pressure, but that the benefit disappeared when subjects consumed a diet that was high in fat, 37 percent of the total calories. So, as is often the case, moderation is the winning ticket.

The same goes for protein. Harvard University investigators have determined that we need a healthy balance of fats, carbohydrates, and protein. Not only will adequate amounts of protein provide a greater and more long-lasting feeling of fullness following a meal, but it will also lower blood pressure in people not currently eating enough protein. The Harvard scientists recommend a larger daily protein intake than was previously believed to be optimal, 25 percent rather than 15 percent of one's daily calories.

It's no wonder that men and women get frustrated when dietary recommendations change, but the scientific process takes time. The good news is that while some tweaking of the diet might still happen in the future, we've pretty much got it nailed when it comes to knowing what to eat and what not to eat to keep our hearts healthy.

The Lyon Diet Heart Study gave us the first solid proof of the benefits of the Mediterranean diet in reducing heart disease. French researchers compared that diet, rich in olive oil, nuts, olives, avocados, and seafood, with the kind of diet typically prescribed by cardiologists in the United States, the United Kingdom, Australia, and elsewhere, which cut way back on fat, while replacing the fat calories with carbohydrates. The subjects were patients who had suffered heart attacks within the past six months.

Benefits of the Mediterranean diet started to show up after just a year. After twenty-seven months, patients on that dietary program had a significantly lower rate of subsequent heart attacks, other heart problems, and deaths. A follow-up analysis nearly four years later demonstrated the long-term advantages. Imagine that enjoying a diet rich in olive oil and other delicious foods actually saved lives!

Italian doctors in the GISSI-Prevention Study had the same happy results when heart attack patients tried the Mediterranean diet, this time supplemented with omega-3 fatty acids. After three and a half years, the rates of nonfatal heart attacks, strokes, and deaths were down substantially.

The Lyon and GISSI-Prevention studies are particularly noteworthy because their subjects already had heart disease severe enough to have caused heart attacks. If those approaches worked for already diseased men and women, think of what they can do for you!

For example, doctors at the University of Minnesota worked with more than 4,300 healthy young men and women between eighteen and thirty years old at the start and tracked them for fifteen years. People eating the most fruits and vegetables in their diets, as compared with the meat-and-potatoes eaters, had the lowest rates of developing elevated blood pressure. But that doesn't mean they gorged on plant foods. The participants were divided into five groups based on fruit and vegetable consumption, from lowest to highest. Compared with the lowest intake, people in the second-lowest to the highest intake had 27 to 36 percent less likelihood of their blood pressure rising to at least 130/85. So even a little extra effort along these lines can provide a big payoff.

The biggest of all the studies done thus far involves the DASH diet, standing for Dietary Approaches to Stop Hypertension, which was begun in the mid-1900s. It was a major undertaking of the U.S. National Institutes of Health, with 459 men and women participating as volunteers in several medical centers around the world. The DASH diet includes lots of fruits, vegetables, whole grains, seafood, and nonfat and low-fat dairy foods.

The diet worked. Blood pressure fell by an average of 5.5 systolic points and 3.0 diastolic points. Blacks responded with drops of 6.9

and 3.3 points. In people with blood pressure levels higher than 140/90, results were even better, with numbers falling by 11.4 and 5.5 points, respectively. Cholesterol levels also improved by 7 percent.

Medical researchers wondered which would be better for diabetic patients: a high-carb, low-fat diet or a diet higher in monounsaturated fats from foods and oils? The high-carb, low-fat diet actually tended to raise systolic and diastolic blood pressure 6 and 7 mm Hg, respectively, for the forty-two type 2 diabetes subjects, while the higher-fat diet lowered both systolic and diastolic blood pressure by 3 to 4 points after a fourteen-week period.

Why does this sort of diet work so well? One theory is that a diet rich in fruits, vegetables, and nonfat and low-fat dairy foods might work as a natural diuretic, much as do certain drugs that are prescribed for lowering blood pressure. These medications have been used to fight hypertension for decades. It's still unknown whether the blood pressure effects gotten from the diet are the result of a specific food or foods or a combination of all of them. The diet is rich in potassium and calcium, both of which help the body to eliminate sodium in the urine. Yet apparently there's more to it than that because supplementation with those two minerals doesn't yield as strong a result.

Another reason the diet lowers blood pressure, some scientists believe, might be due to the effects of plant protein as compared with animal protein. The INTERMAP study involved 4,680 men and women from the United States, the United Kingdom, Japan, and China, representing seventeen diverse populations. Consumption of animal protein didn't affect blood pressure, but plant protein intake was significantly correlated with lower blood pressure.

So many studies have shown the enormous benefits of consuming omega-3 fatty acids from both fish and supplements. They have a powerful influence on improving blood pressure and have many other advantages for heart health.

But, hey, who really cares *why* these sorts of diets work? The important thing is that they do!

At least one study has shown that patients with mildly elevated blood pressure can bring their levels down with this diet alone. For individuals who need prescription drugs, the diet can reduce their necessary dosages. But the best news is that combining this dietary approach, modified to suit one's personal tastes and food preferences, with the newly proven supplementation detailed in this book, eliminates the need for prescription drugs for all but the most severe cases of hypertension.

Whichever part or parts of the diet provide the heart-saving benefits, we know for sure that fruits and vegetables are essential and have been proved to slash the risk of stroke. Doctors in Australia and England, reporting in the British journal *The Lancet*, combined the data from multiple studies involving more than a quarter million subjects over a course of thirteen years on average. Compared with people who ate less than three fruit and vegetable servings daily, men and women who consumed three to five had 11 percent less risk of having strokes, and those who gobbled more than five servings had their stroke risk tumble by 26 percent.

Combining wise dietary choices with other lifestyle improvements, such as exercising, controlling your weight, and giving up cigarette smoking, pays off even higher dividends. In an ongoing U.S. study involving thousands of nurses that was conducted through Harvard University, scientists have calculated that fully 82 percent of heart disease events could potentially be prevented. For nonsmokers, further lifestyle modifications could slash their risk by 74 percent. Studies around the globe have demonstrated a similar protection.

So what, exactly, does the Mediterranean diet consist of and how is it different from the average Western diet? Actually, it's more a complete lifestyle that begins with enjoying regular physical activity and wine in moderation (although other forms of alcoholic beverages probably provide similar if not identical protection). Daily foods include eight servings of whole-grain breads and cereals, six servings of vegetables, three of fruit, two of dairy, and just about all the olive oil you would want, short of an amount that would cause you to gain weight. On a weekly basis, there would be five to six servings of fish and seafood; four of poultry; three to four of olives, nuts, and beans; three of potatoes; three of eggs; and three of sweets. A strict Mediterranean diet would allow only four servings of red meat, although, as we'll see, there's room for variations and modifications to suit one's own tastes and preferences.

What about those fruits and vegetables? Are huge amounts recommended by advocates of the Mediterranean diet and eaten by people in Greece, Spain, Italy, and elsewhere in that part of the world? Not really, when you take a closer look at just what a serving size is.

An average serving of fruit is 80 grams (a little less than 3 ounces) and that of vegetables 77 grams. This would be one average apple, a half banana, a half cup of applesauce, two tablespoons of raisins, or a 6-ounce (200 ml) glass of juice. A serving of cooked vegetables is a half-cup. For raw veggies, it's one cup. Or it could be a glass of tomato, carrot, or another vegetable juice.

How might that fit into an average day? For breakfast you might start with a glass of juice. Then slice half a banana into your cereal or add one-fourth cup of blueberries or another fruit. At your midmorning and midafternoon breaks, try to replace the coffee and the doughnut with a glass of juice or a piece of fruit, at least two or three days a week. Keep a ready supply of dried fruits for snacks at home, in the car, and where you work.

Most of us are far too busy to do much in the way of making lunch. Without planning, this can result in urgent hunger that you satisfy with high-calorie, high-fat, low-nutrient fast food. Here's a suggestion for something faster: soup. A nice steaming bowl is extremely satisfying and remarkably soothing at midday. Chicken and vegetable, minestrone, lentil, split pea, beef and barley, the list goes on. Either order a bowl at a restaurant or use a microwave to heat up a container you bring from home. You'll get two or three servings of veggies, or even more, in that one meal.

I love the sandwiches sold in Subway shops. I can choose from a nice variety of breads and fillings, from seafood to turkey, to ham, tuna, and many others. And I can get a pile of veggies stuffed into those sandwiches: bell peppers, chilis, olives, onions, tomatoes, and lettuce, all freshly chopped.

For the evening meal, get into the habit of putting two or three different vegetables on the plate. For convenience, keep a variety of frozen veggies in the freezer. They're free of sodium, inexpensive, and just about as nutritious as fresh. Start the meal with a nice salad or a cup of soup. Then for evening snacks, more fruit.

What about cost? One doctor wrote a letter to *The Lancet* pointing out that in Scotland, 48 percent of the population eat fresh fruit once a week or less and 41 percent eat green vegetables once a week or less. He suggested that perhaps it was a matter of economics, but that's just not true. First, at least in most parts of the world, seasonal fruits and vegetables are inexpensive. Second, when fresh is not available, people can buy frozen produce that will provide virtually identical nutritional value. Actually, studies have demonstrated that frozen fruits and vegetables can be higher in nutrients than their fresh counterparts since they are flash frozen almost immediately after harvest, while fresh produce may be days old by the time the fruits and vegetables are picked, boxed, shipped, and sold at retail.

For most people, the problem with fruits and vegetables, to be perfectly honest, is that they are boring. Eating steamed vegetables every night would take the dedication of a monk. Fruit can be more interesting if you shoot for variety, but even then you eventually run out of different kinds. So how do those people in the Mediterranean and elsewhere eat so darned much of the plant foods? They're way more creative. That's why I've provided a lot of ideas about preparation in the following recipe section. And consider some perhaps unusual choices. Pomegranates have been a healthful part of the diets of Middle Eastern and Mediterranean countries for centuries. Several recent studies have demonstrated their protective benefits against heart disease and elevated blood pressure. The crunchy ruby-red seeds burst not only with juicy flavor but also with nutrients, including vitamin C and potassium. Enjoy them as a snack or as a colorful and exotic addition to a salad.

When my children were little, I wanted to instill in them a love of fruits and veggies. But kids aren't any different from adults. They have to really be tempted. Offer a child—or an adult—a bowl of apples, pears, or peaches and you won't get much in the way of excitement.

So when Ross and Jenny came home from school, looking for a snack, I devised some tempting treats. Instead of a whole apple, I sliced that apple and used raisins to make faces. Pretty simple. Other times I sliced a variety of fruits and offered them on a plate with some fruit-flavored yogurt as a dip. When I had the time and wanted to be creative, I cut bell peppers to use as "palm fronds" on "trunks" of longitudinally sliced carrots, perhaps with a "bush" of broccoli, and a "pond" of low-fat salad dressing on a platter. Mothers in the neighborhood began to wonder why their kids wanted to come to our house after school! Yup, I was Mr. Mom, and I loved it.

Again, adults aren't much different from children. Take the time to prepare similar creations for yourself and you'll enjoy those snacks a whole lot more.

Chocolate's Healthy Side

In Woody Allen's comedy film *Sleeper*, doctors in the distant future comment on how hot fudge sundaes were eventually found to be "health food." In a turn suggesting that life does in fact sometimes imitate art, research for the last decade has focused on the heart-health benefits of dark chocolate.

One such report came from the University of L'Aguila in Italy in 2005. Researchers there, in collaboration with doctors at Tufts University in Boston, found that dark chocolate, thanks to its high content of plant substances called flavonoids, lowered blood pressure nicely. They gave patients 100 grams of either dark chocolate or white chocolate daily. The dark confection, but not the white, brought systolic blood pressure down by 11.9 mm Hg and diastolic blood pressure down by 8.5. In fact, the darker the chocolate, the greater the level of those beneficial flavonoids.

Yet eating chocolate every day isn't a realistic approach to blood pressure control. You'd get 580 calories from that 100 gram bar, along with 45 grams of fat, 27.5 grams of which are saturated. Much of the research has been sponsored by the Mars Candy Company, based in Chicago, Illinois. While that company has enjoyed expected headlines in the media, the real purpose of the research is to eventually isolate the specific flavonoids, synthesize the chemicals, and make them available perhaps as a prescription drug for blood pressure. That would be a good thing, since such a "drug" would not be expected to have the adverse effects that drugs on the market now have. But it will be years before that product might hit the pharmacy shelves.

In the meantime, we can all reap the benefits of chocolate without the fat and the calories. Chocolate is made from cocoa, butter, cocoa butter, and sugar. The healthy flavonoids are in the cocoa. So enjoy cocoa in a variety of delicious ways, including hot cocoa and the desserts detailed in the recipe section in chapter 17. Buy pure cocoa powder, not the instant mixes that also contain sugar and fat, to get the most of both flavonoids and flavor.

Coffee, Tea, Cola, and Your Heart

How do you start your day? Most men and women get going with a cup of either coffee or tea. Your choice may well be having an impact on your heart health in general and your blood pressure in particular.

In 2005, a long-term study that tracks the lifestyles and the health of nearly 156,000 nurses provided some insights. Harvard researchers compared coffee and cola consumption with development of hypertension over a twelve-year period. Habitual coffee drinking wasn't associated with increased blood pressure, but cola sodas, both diet and regular, were. Digging further into the data, I discovered that women consuming the most caffeine, whether from coffee or cola, were at no greater risk than those with the lowest intake. Why, then, might cola beverages pose some risk? That'll be determined, we hope, by further research.

In the meantime, however, it appears that coffee drinkers can breathe a sigh of relief and enjoy their beverage of choice in moderation. Conversely, it might be a good idea to limit cola drinking and perhaps to switch off now and then with other flavors of soda.

An exception for coffee drinkers came from work done by Swiss investigators, who found that drinking two cups of caffeinated coffee decreases blood flow to the heart during exercise, especially at high altitudes. On a practical level, it seems that we should keep coffee drinking to just one cup before exercise and avoid it entirely while climbing or hiking in the mountains.

So much for blood pressure, but what about coffee and cholesterol? There have been mixed reports, and many consumers are justifiably confused. It is true that coffee can elevate levels of the harmful LDL cholesterol, but only when prepared in either the French or the Scandinavian styles. Using a French press coffee maker or dumping ground coffee beans into boiling water, it appears, releases two chemicals called diterpenes that are wholly responsible for LDL increases. Drip coffee making, which does not squeeze the grounds or use boiling hot water, has no ill effects on cholesterol. Decaf drinkers aren't completely out of the woods. If your brew is made from robusta rather than Arabica beans, decaf coffee can, unfortunately, raise LDL counts. Robusta beans, which are less expensive than the Arabica type, are often used in decaf since they are stronger and provide more flavor following the decaffeination process. It may well be worth the small extra expense to opt for buying decaf made with Arabica beans.

If your beverage of choice happens to be tea, smile when you take the next sip. Or you might even consider switching from coffee to tea after reading this. While coffee, at best, does no harm, tea can provide great benefit in terms of heart health. More than a decade of research has shown us that tea drinkers suffer less heart disease. Chinese investigators in Taiwan have quantified those benefits.

They examined the long-term effects of tea drinking on the development of hypertension and found that the more tea consumed, the lower the risk. The doctors recruited more than 1,500 men and women ages twenty years or older who had no history of elevated blood pressure levels. They then tracked how much tea the subjects drank and how many of them developed hypertension. People who drank 120 to 599 ml of tea daily showed a 46 percent decrease in risk, as compared with individuals who typically drink less than 120 ml a day. The more, the better. People gulping 600 ml or more daily cut their risk by a whopping 65 percent. When the investigators looked at tea consumption over a ten-year, rather than a one-year, period of time, they found no additional benefit. In other words, the benefit continued but did not increase.

Those nice benefits are restricted to real tea, not herbal types. It doesn't seem to matter whether tea is decaf or regular, but most tea drinkers of the world consume regular, full-strength tea. On a practical level, bear in mind that tea contains theobromine, the chemical cousin of caffeine, and drinking large quantities can jangle the nerves just as coffee can. Seek moderation in all things.

Fish, Supplements, and the Search for Heart-Healthy Omega-3 Fatty Acids

Seldom are research findings unequivocal. Usually, you can find data to defend both sides of a debate. Omega-3 fatty acids are the exception to the rule. The more scientists investigate the way fish oils work in the body, the more benefits they find, with virtually no negatives to report.

Initially, of course, we heard about the Inuit Eskimos of Greenland and how they almost never developed heart disease even though they ate large amounts of fat in the form of fish and marine animals. At first glance, that appeared paradoxical. Then came the realization that the fat consumed was a kind of polyunsaturated fatty acid termed omega-3. Think about it: if the fat in coldwater fish were saturated, those fish would be as stiff and hard as a stick of butter in the refrigerator.

Next was a long-term study of workers at the Western Electric Company in Chicago, hinting that fish lovers enjoyed protection against heart disease. The risk of a fatal heart attack was slashed by a third just from this one lifestyle factor. A similar investigation that examined the habits of tens of thousands of male physicians revealed that those who ate fish at least once a week had half the risk of sudden cardiac death.

The list of research studies goes on and on, all with favorable results. We now know that the main fish oils, eicosapentanoic acid (EPA) and docohexanoic acid (DHA), work in a number of wonderful ways. These omega-3 fatty acids reduce the formation of blood clots and raise levels of the protective HDL cholesterol while dramatically lowering triglycerides. They prevent heart rhythm disturbances and they lower heart rates. Because heart rate is associated with the risk of sudden death, this association may at least partially explain the lower risk of sudden death among people who regularly eat fish.

A fairly new observation shows the ability of omega-3 fatty acids to lower blood pressure. They appear to do so by reducing resistance to surges of blood flow in the arteries. That, in turn, improves performance of the left ventricle of the heart, the muscular pump. What we have, as a result, is healthier arteries that are less stiff and more flexible, as well as a more powerful heart muscle, both of which improve blood flow and hence reduce blood pressure.

Both fish and fish oil supplements providing the omega-3 fatty acids EPA and DHA have been clinically documented to yield these benefits for the heart and the vascular system. It turns out that even small amounts of fish, especially the fatty, coldwater fish such as salmon, herring, sardines, and mackerel, do the trick. One needn't eat fish daily, giving up all other meats. The American Heart Association recommends having two fish meals weekly. That's solidly backed up in the medical literature.

I happen to be one of those lucky guys who really loves fish. In restaurants, I most frequently order salmon, not just because it's good for me but because I simply enjoy it, whether grilled, roasted, blackened, or poached. For a little snack to tide me over before dinner I'll have herring, either pickled or creamed, on whole-wheat crackers. Smoked salmon, also known as lox, on a bagel with a smear of low-fat cream cheese? That's heaven to me!

But not everyone likes, much less loves, fish. For them, supplements are the answer. After many years of experimentation most authorities now agree on the optimal dosage. If you're buying fish oil capsules, shoot for 3 grams daily. You can also get the omega-3 fats EPA and DHA in a concentrated ethyl ester form, in which case you'd need only 1 gram a day. People using omega-3 supplements to reduce very high levels of triglyderides will require 3.5 grams daily; that dosage is considered pharmacological, acting like a drug, and should be taken under medical supervision.

You may hear about getting omega-3s from plant sources, especially flaxseed and flaxseed oil but also from soybeans, canola and walnut oils, and various kinds of nuts. All of those foods contain a far less potent form of the beneficial fatty acids called alpha-linolenic acid (ALA). You may even see ALA supplements on sale in health food stores and pharmacies, but only a fraction, a small fraction, of ALA is converted by the body into EPA and DHA. Stick with the fish oils or the concentrated ethyl ester supplements.

There is only one broad contraindication. Patients taking the potent blood-thinning drug Coumadin (warfarin) by prescription from their physicians should not, under any circumstances, take omega-3 supplements. If you take those drugs, talk with your doctor about the safe consumption of fish meals.

What about the mercury contamination of fish? It's true that mercury, a heavy metal, becomes concentrated in the fatty tissues of fish. That's particularly true for tilefish, swordfish, king mackerel, and shark, all of which contain 1 part per million or more of mercury. But, as reported in the November 28, 2002, issue of the *New England Journal of Medicine*, many if not most fish do not have appreciable amounts. Fresh and frozen tuna have 0.32 parts per million (ppm) and canned tuna drops down to 0.17 ppm. Pollack has 0.20 ppm. In both salmon and shrimp, mercury is not detectable.

Certainly, the small amounts of mercury in fish other than those with 1 or more ppm do not pose a threat, and the benefits to heart health far outweigh any potential risk. Pregnant women and small children, however, should limit their consumption of fish varieties that are higher in the heavy metal. As with all such matters, discuss this with your physician.

OMEGA-3 FATTY ACID CONTENT OF FISH
(GRAM/3 OZ SERVING)

Sardines (Norway)	5.1	Bluefish	1.2
Sockeye salmon	2.7	Mackerel (Pacific)	1.1
Mackerel (Atlantic)	2.5	Striped bass	0.8
King salmon	1.9	Yellowfin tuna	0.6
Herring	1.7	Pollock	0.5
Lake trout	1.4	Brook trout	0.4
Albacore tuna	1.3	Yellow perch	0.3
Halibut	1.3	Catfish	0.2

For the most part, people tend to eat and enjoy the foods they grew up with. It's stating the obvious to say that French people like French food, Italians love Italian dishes, and people living in China prefer not only Chinese food but specifically the preparations from the province of their birth. Although I like Chinese food, after a month's stay in that country, I was really tired of it.

I've always thought that those of us who live in the United States, Canada, the United Kingdom, Australia, and other countries with large immigrant populations are lucky to have ready access to a wide variety of cuisines from all over the world. One day it can be Italian, the next day Greek, the day after that Chinese or Thai or Japanese, and on it goes. Moreover, we have our own regional preferences.

Growing up in the Midwest, I developed and still have a strong affinity for meatloaf with mashed potatoes and gravy. The English invented shepherd's pie, and Englishmen eat it throughout their lives. In Australia, it's the beloved meat pies.

So does it mean that you must abandon those sorts of preferences in order to benefit your blood pressure readings? Must you eat nothing but Greek food as prepared on the shores of the Mediterranean to follow a "Mediterranean" diet? Nothing could be further from the truth. One scientific investigation, for example, was titled the Indo-Mediterranean Diet Heart Study, reflecting the influences of Indian cuisine. Next, consider how many very different countries surround the Mediterranean Sea. I'm looking at a map as I write this, noting, beyond the obvious Italy and Greece, countries such as Morocco, Algeria, Tunisia, France, Turkey, Croatia, Albania, and the vast expanse of Middle Eastern countries: Egypt, Israel, Syria, Lebanon, and others. And don't forget the foods of the Far East, which have also been noted for their heart-healthy qualities. Their national cuisines are very different but have certain things in common: lots of fruits and vegetables, plenty of fish and seafood, poultry, low-fat red meats (including some you might not find in your market, such as goat, water buffalo, and camel), whole-grain breads and cereals, and foods and oils rich in monounsaturated fatty acids.

Moreover, and probably most important of all, we can tweak the favored dishes of our origins to bring down saturated fats and increase monounsaturated fats and vegetables. Yes, even meatloaf, shepherd's pie, and meat pie. Olive oil is not necessarily the panacea, the only choice you have. There's also canola oil, which is rich in monounsaturated fats and extremely low in saturated fats. Other oils fill the bill as well. Let me give you one example before I describe a treasure trove of heart-healthy, cholesterol-lowering, and blood pressure–improving recipes. I really enjoy chili con carne, as do most Americans. But my version today includes two cans of chili beans instead of one to boost the level of plant protein and soluble fiber, ground beef that's very low in fat, low-sodium canned tomatoes, and a can of chili peppers. I like to sprinkle on grated low-fat cheddar cheese and mellow the chili with a dollop of low-fat sour cream. Wine just doesn't pair well with chili, so it's always a bottle of beer. Nothing like that was ever served in Greece or Italy, although they have somewhat similar dishes, but it has all the heart-healthy attributes of the Mediterranean diet even though it had its origins along the Texas/Mexico border.

Assuming that you love food as much as I do, I'm delighted to share some dishes from the Kowalski cookbook with you in the recipes and suggestions I offer in chapter 17.

13

Daily Blood Pressure Busters

We know for certain that blood pressure tends to rise as we get older. Family history plays a big role. Elevated blood pressure, in turn, raises our risk of having strokes and heart attacks. While there's not much we can do to turn back the hands of time and we can't choose our parents and grandparents, there are also a lot of things that appear to lower blood pressure and the risk of developing cardiovascular disease. Conversely, there are other things, some of which are touted in magazines and health food stores, that have little or no effect or may even raise blood pressure. Perversely, some medications, both over-the-counter and prescription-only, can make blood pressure go up.

Rather than appear to give priority to one or the other in my review of these things, I've chosen to discuss them in alphabetical order. It's a real potpourri of ideas you may never have heard of or considered.

Acupuncture and Blood Pressure

This Asian technique has been used for centuries by Chinese, Japanese, and Korean physicians to treat a wide variety of ailments. In 2005, German researchers reported their findings on the effectiveness of acupuncture in the treatment of high blood pressure at the annual scientific sessions of the American Heart Association.

They worked with 160 male and female patients ages forty-five to seventy-five, all of whom had mild to moderate hypertension. Seventy-eight percent were taking antihypertensive drugs. During a six-week trial, patients were given either acupuncture or a sham treatment designed to appear the same as acupuncture.

Of that starting group, 141 patients completed the trial; 72 got acupuncture and 69 received the sham treatment or placebo. Immediately after the subjects received acupuncture, their blood pressure fell from an average of 131/81 to 125/78, but the sham treatment had no impact during a twenty-four-hour period. When patients were tested three and six months later, however, there were no residual effects from the acupuncture treatment.

Unless you happen to live with an acupuncture therapist, this doesn't seem to be a practical way to control blood pressure.

Aspirin and Blood Pressure

Native Americans, the people Christopher Columbus called "Indians," were peeling off the bark of willow trees and drinking a tea brewed from it to ease their aches and pains long before Europeans set foot in the New World. Eventually, the active ingredient was isolated and identified as acetylsalicylic acid, more commonly known as aspirin. In 1899, Bayer launched a synthesized aspirin product as an anti-inflammatory and painkilling over-the-counter medicine, and it quickly became the most widely used agent in the history of medicine.

In 1960, researchers found that aspirin has an "antiplatelet" activity; it keeps blood cells called platelets from forming clots. Today the U.S. Food and Drug Administration and other regulatory agencies throughout the world approve aspirin to reduce the risk of having a stroke, for immediate treatment of a possible heart attack, and to prevent second heart attacks. A study of fifty-five thousand patients showed that daily aspirin can prevent a first heart attack in apparently healthy individuals, reducing their risk by 32 percent.

It's a good thing that no one pharmaceutical manufacturer has an exclusive patent on the stuff, or we'd be paying through the nose! Aspirin is one of the cheapest ways to protect our hearts.

Of course, like almost anything else, aspirin can cause problems in certain individuals. It raises the risk of gastrointestinal bleeding and a type of stroke termed *hemorrhagic*, in which bleeding occurs in the brain. But those adverse reactions are relatively rare, and the risk/benefit ratio is very good.

A meta-analysis of six trials involving a total of more than ninety-five thousand men and women was performed and published in 2006. Researchers concluded that aspirin reduced the risk of strokes in women and heart attacks in men. Overall, women taking low dosages of aspirin had a 12 percent lower risk of suffering either a heart attack, a stroke, or a cardiovascular disease–related death. Postmenopausal women and those who had suffered a previous cardiovascular event experienced the most benefit. Men enjoyed a 14 percent reduction in risk.

Doctors typically recommend a low-dose 81 mg aspirin tablet daily. Some studies have shown effectiveness with 100 mg every other day. Taking a coated tablet can lessen gastric upset and potential bleeding, but some studies have indicated lesser protection because of the coating. Preliminary observations show that the optimum time to take one's daily aspirin would be at bedtime rather than in the morning, since it reduces levels of nocturnal blood pressure, though not daytime blood pressure.

Breathing and Blood Pressure

Unlike dolphins and other animals who must make a conscious effort to breathe, humans are "autobreathers" who don't give it a thought. Well, we should do so. It turns out that when we breathe rapidly and shallowly, our blood pressure goes up. Conversely, when we slow down our breathing rate and deliberately breathe deeply both in and out, we can make our blood pressure go down.

If you have decided to purchase a blood pressure monitor, which I discussed in chapter 2, try this simple test. Walk rapidly to wherever the device is, sit down, start it up, and measure your blood pressure. Jot down the numbers. Then close your eyes and spend two or three minutes concentrating on your breathing. Very deliberately breathe in deeply, feeling your lungs expanding to the fullest. Hold that breath for a bit. Then slowly, slowly let the air out, and, when you think you're completely deflated like a balloon, puff out the last remaining air. Repeat the process. Again, think about your breathing. Enjoy the feeling of the air fully inflating your lungs and finally deflating. Now retest your pressure. Almost certainly it'll be lower. Now do another session of deliberate and slow breathing before testing the third time. Your blood pressure will be lower still. This is pretty powerful stuff that shows how we have personal control over our bodies.

Is this just a parlor trick that has no lasting effect? If you do it just that one time, yes. But if you make it a habit to take several little mini-vacations a day of deep breathing, eventually you'll see a lasting benefit. You'll eventually reach a point where you breathe fewer times per minute throughout the entire day. How many times per minute do you breathe now? You probably have no idea unless you make it a point to count your breaths. Do so now. Note the number. Then make an effort to breathe fewer times per minute but more fully and deeply. Studies have proven that people who do this will have lower blood pressure levels.

There is a device on the market to help you achieve the goal of blood pressure reduction through improved breathing. Aptly named "RESPeRATE," the little machine is about the size of a paperback book and is battery operated; you can take it anywhere. The device automatically analyzes your breathing rate and pattern and interactively guides you through a breathing exercise to slow down your breathing from the normal rate of fourteen to eighteen breaths per minute to the therapeutic zone of less than ten breaths per minute, with prolonged exhalation as I described previously.

At first, breathing returns to normal after each session of RESPeRATE use, but gradually you'll find that your breath-per-minute rate and the depth of your breathing improves. Researchers say that with regular use, the beneficial effects on blood pressure build up to create a lasting blood pressure reduction.

Clinical studies have shown the device to be capable of lowering blood pressure by an average of 14 systolic points and 9 diastolic points after eight weeks of routine use, consisting of fifteen minutes a day three or four times a week. Average reductions, the researchers have found, are greater for older patients and people with higher blood pressure to begin with. Those reductions would be over and above any achieved from other forms of therapy.

For more information on RESPeRATE, go to www.high-blood-pressure-help.com. Can you do it completely on your own without the device? Sure, but it's likely that the greatest benefit will occur with the assistance of this little device. There's also the advantage of relying on a machine as if it were a professional psychologist guiding you through breathing sessions. You'll find this is a wonderful way to deal with stress.

Coenzyme Q10 and Blood Pressure

Coenzyme Q10, or CoQ10, is a substance that occurs naturally in virtually all of our bodies' tissues, especially in muscle tissue. It's so widespread throughout the body that another name for it is ubiquinone, referring to its ubiquitous nature. CoQ10 regulates energy in muscle cells. As we age, the amount in our bodies declines. For that reason, it has been speculated that supplementation would improve energy levels. That claim hasn't been well substantiated, but there are other and better reasons to consider supplementation.

Statin drugs that are prescribed to lower cholesterol also lower the production of CoQ10, sometimes to a point of frank deficiency. That's because statin drugs inhibit an enzyme that's essential for the body's manufacture of both cholesterol and CoQ10. Medical researchers at the University of California at San Diego believe that the CoQ10 depletion caused by statin drugs may be responsible for the drug's potential for causing muscle aches and permanent muscle damage. They recommend CoQ10 supplementation for everyone taking statin drugs.

What about CoQ10 and blood pressure? Researchers theorize that most hypertensive patients have a significant CoQ10 deficiency that in turn leads to a deficiency in a naturally occurring provitamin, a substance that "energizes" and maximizes the potential of vitamins. At least eight trials looked at the effect of varying dosages of CoQ10 on blood pressure. All of them showed benefit, although blood pressure reductions varied.

In one trial, thirty patients received 60 mg of CoQ10 twice daily while a control group of twenty-nine other patients got a B-vitamin placebo for eight weeks. The CoQ10 group had a very nice 16-point drop in systolic blood pressure and a 9-point fall in diastolic pressure. People in that group also had reductions in triglycerides, blood sugar, and insulin, with increases in HDL and serum levels of vitamins A, C, and E. The B-vitamin placebo control group saw only an increase in vitamin C in the blood.

Another study examined the effects of CoQ10 on what's called isolated systolic hypertension in which only the systolic, not the diastolic, pressure is elevated. A group of forty-six men and thirty-seven women got either 60 mg of CoQ10 daily or a placebo for twelve weeks. People taking the CoQ10 had decreases in systolic blood pressure from 10.5 to a whopping 25.1, with an average of 17.8. That's wonderful, but not all studies have shown such dramatic improvements.

Part of the reason for the variance in effectiveness of CoQ10 may come down to whether a person has a low level of the substance in the tissues and the bloodstream to begin with. You could take a test to measure your CoQ10 levels, or you could simply undertake a two- or three-month trial to see what sort of benefit it might provide. Certainly, there are no possible downsides to CoQ10 supplementation, and you might note an improvement in energy as well as a decrease in blood pressure. It might work for you and it might not, but there's no reason not to try it.

Eye Examinations and Blood Pressure

Now, what could eye exams possibly have to do with blood pressure, you might reasonably ask? Well, it turns out that the eyes may be the window through which to look for potential future hypertension. The little arterioles that supply blood to the retina apparently get narrower before blood pressure elevations proceed to hypertension; an eye doctor can spot the narrowing before blood pressure goes up at all. An investigation in Sydney, Australia, called the Blue Mountain Eye Study found that people with narrowed blood vessels in the eyes were twice as likely as people with normal arterioles to develop hypertension over a five-year period. Those predictions of hypertension were independent of other factors, including smoking, weight, and even blood pressure levels at the start of the study.

The retinas of the 3,654 Sydney residents who participated in the study were photographed with special cameras. Participants were mostly forty-nine years old or older. While the changes in the retinal arterioles predicted hypertension regardless of age, the association was strongest for people younger than sixty-five.

This study confirmed the findings of another project, the Atherosclerosis Risk in Communities Study, which found that retinal blood vessel narrowing predicted hypertension within three years. Doctors point out that by knowing the risk of future blood pressure problems, one can immediately take lifestyle modification steps to avoid them.

Hypertension is also more prevalent in patients with glaucoma, according to researchers in England who worked with more than twenty-seven thousand subjects who had the eye disease. Doctors in that study speculate that sodium retention may be the underlying cause of both glaucoma and hypertension.

Conversely, controlling blood pressure may be a way to prevent glaucoma. Investigators at the University of Wisconsin found that decreases in blood pressure are associated with reduced pressure in the eye, intraocular pressure. Since intraocular pressure is said to be the most important risk factor for glaucoma, treating blood pressure levels before they reach the hypertension stages may first reduce intraocular pressure and subsequently prevent both hypertension and glaucoma. There was a direct and linear association between rises in blood pressure and increases in intraocular pressure.

Fermented Milk and Blood Pressure

People in Scandinavia love fermented milk and enjoy it frequently as a beverage. Fermented milk is sold in several European countries. Good for them, because that fermented milk appears to reduce blood pressure. And good for us, since the same bacteria, *Lactobacillus*, that are present in fermented milk are also found in active-culture yogurt that we can find in our food stores.

How do those bacteria help to control blood pressure? The *Lactobacilli* break down the milk protein casein into two types of protein fragments termed *tripeptides*. (Isoleucine/praline/praline and valine/praline/praline for nutritionists and others who might want to know.) Those tripeptides, in turn, block the blood pressure–raising, kidney-derived enzyme called angiotensin-converting enzyme (ACE). You might find that to be a mouthful, but you may well have heard about ACE inhibitors, which are antihypertensive prescription drugs. So the milk tripeptides work the same way as the powerful ACE inhibitor drugs.

Finnish researchers worked with ninety-four study participants who had hypertension and were not taking antihypertensive drugs. They got either 150 ml of fermented milk or a control beverage twice daily for ten weeks. The milk reduced their systolic pressure by an average of 4 points and the diastolic pressure by 2 points. An insignificant improvement, you sniff? Studies have shown that a 3-point reduction in systolic blood pressure cuts one's stroke risk by 10 to 13 percent and the chances of having a heart attack by 7 percent. That's very significant.

If you're a yogurt lover, make sure to look for products whose labels declare "active cultures." If you enjoy yogurt twice a day— say, with breakfast and for a snack—you might be able to get your blood pressure down quite a bit.

Fish Oil and Blood Pressure

We know for certain that people who eat fish, especially coldwater fatty fish such as salmon, herring, and sardines, protect themselves against cardiovascular disease. But can fish oil supplements provide similar protection? Specifically, can taking those supplements help to control blood pressure?

The fish fats that appear to convey heart-healthly benefits are the omega-3 fatty acids EPA and DHA. Their potential for lowering blood pressure comes through modulating calcium ions inside cells of the body, which signals arterial smooth muscles to dilate, thus narrowing the lumen, the opening, of the artery and raising blood pressure. The mode of action, then, would be similar to the calcium channel blocker category of antihypertensive drugs.

Studies have indeed shown a blood pressure–lowering effect of fish oil supplementation. But dosages have been very high, to a point that one would develop "fish breath" and burping, thus limiting compliance.

Conversely, supplementation with 1,000 mg of EPA/DHA (either in purified capsules that concentrate the EPA/DHA or in about 3,000 mg of fish oil, which is needed to provide that amount of EPA/DHA) conveys a number of heart-healthly benefits, including a reduction of triglyceride levels, improved HDL, and lessened blood clotting. That dosage would not typically cause the side effects noted previously. Would such supplementation improve your blood pressure? It's worth trying if you don't already enjoy fish at least two or three days a week; if you do eat fish regularly, you'll get those other benefits anyway.

Personally, I'm one of the lucky people who really loves fish of all sorts, so I don't take any fish oil supplements. I'm more likely to order fish than meat in a restaurant, and I enjoy snacking on herring and crackers pretty regularly.

Do not take fish oil supplements of any kind if you are currently taking the drugs heparin or Plavix. Both of those drugs lessen the body's ability to form blood clots. Taking fish oils (omega-3 fatty acids) could make clotting capabilities lower than your doctor would want. Speak with him or her about this if you are taking these or other "blood-thinner" drugs.

Folic Acid and Blood Pressure

Folic acid is one of the B vitamins. Research has established that consuming about 800 micrograms by way of foods and supplements, along with vitamins B6 and B12, reduces levels of the amino acid homocysteine, another risk factor for heart disease. Now recent findings demonstrate that folic acid can also protect against hypertension and the risk of strokes.

In an ongoing study with more than ninety-three thousand female nurses, tracking all aspects of their lifestyles, including diet and physical activity, women who consumed 800 micrograms or more of folic acid daily had a 29 percent lower risk of developing high blood pressure than did women whose intake was less than 200 micrograms a day. The lead investigator, Dr. John Forman of Boston's Brigham and Women's Hospital, said there is evidence that folic acid has a direct effect on the health of the blood vessels. Most of the women in the study who consumed high levels of folic acid took supplements; it's difficult to get 800 micrograms or more from food alone. That amount would be found in any daily vitamin/mineral supplement plus a B-complex supplement.

Another study, from the Baker Heart Research Institute in Melbourne, Australia, showed that folic acid supplementation for just three weeks reduces both blood pressure in the brachial artery of the arm and arterial stiffness. The investigators concluded that "Folic acid is a safe and effective supplement that targets large artery stiffness and may prevent isolated systolic hypertension."

Researchers in Sweden found that individuals eating a diet rich in green leafy vegetables, dried beans, and other vegetables and fruits had a reduced risk of having hemorrhagic strokes. They found a strong connection between levels of folate, the form of the B vitamin found in foods, in the blood and the chances of suffering that type of stroke. They did not see a difference in the risk of the more common type of stroke termed *ischemic*, which is caused by blockage of the carotid arteries providing blood and oxygen to the brain. Perhaps that's because it would be difficult if not impossible to reach the protective amount of folic acid, 800 micrograms, noted in the other studies without supplementation.

Garlic and Blood Pressure

Proving that garlic keeps vampires away would be very difficult, since one would have to first find some vampires in order to do a scientific study. It appears that proving the benefits of garlic is just as difficult, since one can find data supporting either side of the argument.

The Natural Medicines Comprehensive Database, maintained by the U.S. National Institutes of Health, lists garlic as possibly effective when taken orally for hypertension. A meta-analysis, combining the data from many trials, showed that garlic decreases systolic blood pressure by an average of 7.7 points and diastolic pressure by 5.0 points when compared with a placebo. But some placebo-controlled studies have shown no such benefit, and positive studies have been small and uncontrolled. Maybe the differences are owing to variances in the formulation or the type of garlic powder supplement studied. The Kyolic brand seems to be the best, as judged by studies showing a positive effect.

Yet most authorities would agree that using fresh, natural garlic cloves in cooking is a healthy thing to do. Fresh garlic cells contain the amino acid alliin, considered to be the most active garlic constituent. When those cells are broken, as in crushing or mincing the cloves, alliin is converted to allicin by the enzyme allinase. It appears that the allicin is effective in the treatment of hypertension by causing smooth muscle relaxation in arteries, as well as vasodilation, the widening of those arteries, allowing a freer flow of blood upon demand.

So, if you enjoy garlic in your food, you've got some pretty good justification. It may not keep away vampires, but it could drive some extra health into your heart. Just make sure that the people you're with share that garlic with you or your breath will keep them away as if they were vampires.

Herbs and Blood Pressure

Many of my readers automatically assume that I'm an advocate of herbal remedies because I favor natural approaches to health. Theoretically, the use of herbs makes a lot of sense. They have been used for millennia all over the world. A number of widely prescribed drugs began as botanicals, including aspirin from willow tree bark and digitalis, the heart medicine, from the foxglove plant. All well and good. But buying herbs is like buying the proverbial pig in a poke. You have no idea of the purity or the concentration of the active ingredients. Other than in Germany, governments provide little or no regulation. You just don't know what you're getting and taking into your body, and that poses the potential of causing harm as much as benefit.

One study found that twelve of fourteen herbal remedies marketed as treatments for hypertension actually raised blood pressure. Examples include ginkgo, ginseng, licorice, and St. John's wort. Other herbs just don't do anything for blood pressure at all. Take the study of hawthorn, an herb used for years, especially in Europe, for the treatment of heart failure and touted as an antihypertensive agent. Subjects entered one of four groups and received hawthorn (500 mg of the hawthorn leaf extract), magnesium (600 mg), a combination of both, or a placebo. At the end of a ten-week period there was no difference in blood pressure in any of the four groups. Magnesium, by the way, appears to be effective only when included in an effort to balance *all* the electrolytes, which include calcium and potassium, to offset the effects of sodium, as explained in chapter 9.

Laughter and Blood Pressure

This is one of my personal favorites. To me, there's nothing like a good laugh to "cure what ails you," and there's good research to support the idea that laughter can lower your blood pressure. In fact, the latest data indicate that it might be as good for your heart as running or jogging is. (But you should really do both.)

How does laughter work? Maybe it counters the ill effects of stress hormones such as adrenaline and cortisol on blood vessel function. Or perhaps it boosts the body's production of nitric oxide, which relaxes the arterial lining and allows for more efficient blood flow. Both modes of action would in turn lower blood pressure. I think it works in a number of ways, those two and others as well.

A study done at the University of Maryland Medical Center in Baltimore involved healthy men and women whose blood flow through the brachial arteries in their arms was measured noninvasively. Doctors use the brachial artery frequently in this sort of research because dilation in the artery accurately indicates blood flow to and from the heart, and arterial dilation improvement leads to blood pressure lowering.

Measurements were taken before and after the subjects watched either a comedy, *There's Something about Mary*, or a serious, sad film, *Saving Private Ryan*. The researchers found blood vessel dilation to be about 50 percent better on average after the comedy compared with the serious movie.

I don't own a huge collection of DVDs, but comedies make up a large percentage. No one has yet to quantify laughter with blood pressure control. Do you need to watch a comedy or listen to some good stand-up jokes on a daily basis? Is one form of humor better than another? To me, it doesn't matter. There are some things in life you just know are good for you, and having a good belly laugh regularly is one of them.

Loneliness and Blood Pressure

Here we come to the flip side of the emotional coin. If laughter has benefit for the heart, one could suppose that loneliness would have the opposite effect. Indeed, an ever-growing body of evidence suggests that negative energy, whether in the form of anger, hostility, or depression, has a nasty effect on heart health. Harvard research linked loneliness in men with higher levels of arterial inflammation than occurred in men who were not lonely. A study at Duke University found an increased risk of death from heart disease in individuals who were isolated from human contact. One of the latest studies links loneliness to high blood pressure.

In people over the age of fifty who were studied at the University of Chicago, the loneliest people had blood pressure readings as much as 30 points higher than those who weren't lonely. The lonelier the subjects were, the higher their blood pressure readings. Researchers concluded that loneliness can be as bad for the heart as being overweight or sedentary. One could well imagine that lonely men and women would also tend to be overweight as a result of indulging in consolation eating and sedentary, perhaps owing to a lack of companions to engage in physical activity with.

Earlier research suggests that as many as 11 million Americans over age fifty often feel isolated, left out, or lacking in companionship.

The next stage of research will be to determine the potential benefit, as measured by blood pressure, of reducing loneliness. But don't wait for the findings to get published. If you feel that you're one of the lonely, try your utmost to fill the gap in your life. Don't allow yourself to become mired in self-pity or a sense of hopelessness. It's time to make a conscious effort to meet people and possibly make new friends who can provide support and comfort. Build on your own personal likes and loves. Maybe that means volunteering for work through your church or joining like-minded bird lovers for walks in the woods. You could enroll in a sports event such as a bowling team or read to children in schools or the elderly in retirement homes. But, please, do something. There's no reason for any of us to be alone. As human beings, we are naturally social creatures who need the company of others.

Melatonin and Blood Pressure

As our bodies' internal clocks determine that it's time to sleep, triggered largely by the change from daylight to darkness at night, we produce the hormonelike substance melatonin that causes sleepiness. As melatonin levels rise in the blood, blood pressure levels fall during nightly sleep. Italian researchers speculate that melatonin may decrease noradrenaline (norepinephrine) levels, increase nitric oxide production, and lessen the resistance to blood flow within large arteries. All those effects would be expected to lower blood pressure.

So the doctors at a clinic in Modena decided to evaluate the effect of melatonin on the daily blood pressure variance in nine women with normal blood pressure and another nine whose hypertension was being treated with ACE inhibitor drugs. Their ages ranged from forty-seven to sixty-three. For three weeks, the women were randomly assigned to slow-release melatonin (1 mg released rapidly and 2 mg slowly) or a placebo. During the next three weeks, the groups "crossed over" to get melatonin if they had been taking a placebo and vice versa.

Melatonin treatment decreased both systolic and diastolic nightly blood pressure by 3.77 and 3.63 points on average. Some women had as much as a 10-point blood pressure decline during the night's sleep. Women who normally had the least reduction in nocturnal blood pressure showed the greatest improvement.

There was no change in blood pressure during the day, which was to be expected since melatonin levels disappear or diminish after awakening. But the difference between nocturnal and diurnal blood pressure intensified, and that difference has been linked with heart disease. The larger the difference between blood pressure during the day and during the night, the better.

Similar research has been conducted at Harvard University, where investigators gave melatonin to sixteen men over a three-week period. A single dose of 2.5 mg of melatonin did no good, but taken nightly over the course of the three weeks, it reduced systolic and diastolic blood pressure on average by 6 and 4 points, respectively. The difference between blood pressure during the day and during the night was increased by 15 percent systolic and 25 percent diastolic. Subjects enjoyed better sleep as well, although improvement in sleep was not correlated with that of blood pressure.

When I read the first research reports in this area in 2004, I immediately began taking a melatonin tablet every night at bedtime. Why bother if one can't tell any difference since there's no improvement in blood pressure readings during the day? Just as there are typically no symptoms of hypertension, we know it does damage to the arteries and places us at risk of having heart attacks or strokes. And while we can't feel the increased difference between blood pressure at night and during the day, our cardiovascular health will reflect the benefit. Melatonin is exceptionally inexpensive. Why not seek that benefit?

The best product would be a controlled-release melatonin that would keep levels of the substance more constant throughout the hours of sleep. One such choice would be Health Yourself C-R Melatonin, but any time-release, sustained-release, or controlled-release melatonin would be fine.

Music and Blood Pressure

Listening to fast-tempo music tends to increase blood pressure, while slower music may be useful for lowering blood pressure. Random pauses in a piece of music enhance the pressure-lowering effect.

In a collaborative study, researchers from Italy and the United Kingdom played Indian raga, slow classical, fast classical, rap, and modern techno music for twelve classically trained musicians and twelve people with no musical training. Faster-tempo music with simple rhythm patterns increased the breathing rate, the heart rate, and both systolic and diastolic blood pressure. Slower music had less effect, and raga significantly lowered heart rate. During two-minute pauses in the music, the heart rate, blood pressure, and breathing rate decreased even more significantly in both trained and untrained individuals.

This trial appears to contradict other research showing that relaxing, meditative music that is continuous, without pauses, produces lower blood pressure. The researchers speculate that all music has pauses, and that concentrating on the music and then lapsing into pauses may have more of a meditative effect.

Over-the-Counter (OTC) and Prescription Drugs and Blood Pressure

The remedies for allergies, colds, and the occasional flu may play a role in blood pressure elevation that you're not aware of but definitely should be. A meta-analysis of twenty-four placebo-controlled studies involving a total of 1,285 subjects showed a slight blood pressure–raising effect of pseudoephedrine, frequently found in decongestant products or in combination with antihistamines. The effect might be greatest in older individuals and people whose blood pressure is already higher than it should be.

Pain killers and anti-inflammatory agents may also cause a problem. Watch out for acetaminophen (Tylenol), naproxen (OTC Aleve or Rx Naprosyn), and ibuprofen (Advil, Motrin). The prescription-only anti-inflammatory drugs diclofenac (Voltaren) and indomethacin (Indocin) can also increase blood pressure.

Weight-loss products frequently contain stimulants such as bitter orange (*Citrus aurantium*), caffeine, ma huang, and guarana. The use of PPA (phenylpropanolamine) is currently banned in the United States. These substances are meant to depress appetite and to increase energy, thus burning more calories. Often these substances are used in combination, such as caffeine and bitter orange. That particular combination may increase heart rate and blood pressure and create a risk for adverse cardiovascular events, especially for people with existing conditions. Consumerlab.com research determined that two products, LeanSystem 7 and Ripped Fuel, contain the same amount of caffeine as in six and fourteen and a half cans of cola, respectively. All such stimulants, especially in high dosages, have blood pressure–raising potential.

Most younger men and women don't think of energy drinks as drugs, but they contain the same stimulants that are found in certain weight-loss products and have the same potential for raising both heart rate and blood pressure. They also can lead to a risk of dehydration, especially when consumed at parties and clubs while dancing. I agree with many health authorities who believe these energy drinks are a disaster waiting to happen, particularly when used to excess.

"If you have high blood pressure and it's not responding to treatment, it could be because of a medication you're taking," warn doctors at the Mayo Clinic in Rochester, Minnesota. Whether you utilize the nondrug approaches detailed in this book or take prescription antihypertensive drugs or both, be aware that a number of other prescribed drugs can cancel out their blood pressure–lowering potential. These prescription drugs include antidepressants such as bupropion (Wellbutrin, Zyban), anti-inflammatory agents that include celecoxib (Celebrex), and oral contraceptives (OCs). Women older than thirty-five or who are overweight or who drink alcohol more than moderately are at greater risk of developing high blood pressure while taking OCs. Fortunately, most OCs today contain low-level dosages of estrogen, progesterone, or both. Those with more than 50 micrograms of estrogen are most likely to raise blood pressure.

Sleep Disorders and Blood Pressure

We all know how a good night's sleep can make the next day more productive and enjoyable. Doctors also recognize the importance of sleep and how sleep deprivation, common in today's hectic lifestyle, can have a negative impact on health in a number of ways. Perhaps your sleep habits are influencing your blood pressure.

Research from Columbia University in New York links insufficient sleep with elevations in blood pressure. In that study, investigators found that sleeping less than six hours a night more than doubled the risk of developing hypertension. That remained true even after factoring in variables such as obesity and diabetes. Subjects ranged in age from thirty-two to fifty-nine.

Why might getting less-than-recommended amounts of sleep predispose a person to high blood pressure? Pressure levels are lower during sleep than during waking hours. The difference between night and day blood pressure levels protects us against developing hypertension; the greater the difference, subtracting one from the other, the greater the protection. Thus sleeping fewer than the recommended eight hours nightly would expose us to daytime pressures for a longer period of time, and the longer that sleep deprivation, the higher the average pressure will be.

A condition termed *sleep apnea* may be even more deadly. People who suffer with this disorder have difficulty breathing during sleep. Sleep studies have shown patients waking as often as once a minute. This keeps them from ever slipping into a solid, restful sleep. Such individuals actually stop breathing and then abruptly awaken and resume breathing. Snoring, often extremely loud and disturbing to spouses and roommates, is common.

Scientists believe there is a causal link between sleep apnea and hypertension. Alleviating the disorder either by surgically removing tissue that blocks the airway or by pumping air into the nostrils with a machine can lower blood pressure. People suffering from sleep apnea are often obese.

This extreme form of sleep disturbance has also been implicated in causing strokes. Snoring is no laughing matter.

If you suffer from any form of sleep disorder, discuss this fully with your physician as an aspect of controlling your blood pressure.

Vitamin Supplements and Blood Pressure

While there's no question that a diet rich in fruits, vegetables, and whole grains can very effectively lower blood pressure, the same can't be said for vitamin supplements. At the least, clinical trials have come up with mixed results and aren't very encouraging.

Vitamin E appears to have no effect on blood pressure. A randomized, controlled, though open-label (not double-blind, as when neither the researchers nor the subjects know whether they're getting the active agent or a placebo), trial measured blood pressure in 142 patients with controlled hypertension. Giving vitamin E resulted in no change in systolic blood pressure and a small reduction of 1.6 points in diastolic blood pressure.

Vitamin C appears to be more promising. Theoretically, this vitamin functions as an antioxidant that would enhance the synthesis or prevent the breakdown of nitric oxide, a naturally occurring gas produced in the lining of the arteries that keeps those vessels flexible and more capable of vasodilation. Studies have shown reductions in systolic blood pressure though not in diastolic pressure, when subjects were treated with vitamin C. A randomized, placebo-controlled trial with thirty-nine patients yielded nice results. Subjects took a 2 gram "loading dose" and then 500 mg daily for thirty days. Systolic blood pressure was reduced by 13 mm Hg, but vitamin C had no effect on diastolic pressure.

Other trials were not as positive. Moreover, millions of men and women who routinely take at least 500 mg of vitamin C daily and have done so for many years develop hypertension. Supplementation with vitamins C and E may have other benefits, and I think they probably do, but I wouldn't count on either to bring blood pressure down.

14

The Blood Pressure Cure
5 Secret Weapons

More than two decades ago I began my search for ways to lower my own cholesterol levels and prevent an early death from heart disease. Certainly, the essential foundation of such a program had to include increased physical activity and a heart-healthy diet. But knowing that other factors entered into the cholesterol picture—notably, that the body makes 80 percent of all the cholesterol in the bloodstream—I realized that I needed something more than diet and exercise. My search led me to the soluble fibers in oat bran and other foods that actually flush out cholesterol and the vitamin niacin to stop the body's excessive production of it. Since that time, I've found additional natural approaches to lowering cholesterol, including the plant sterols known as phytosterols, red yeast rice, and pantethine.

So it was with a sense of déjà vu that I began my own search to normalize my blood pressure. I've detailed the foundation of a solid program in the chapters of this book, and these lifestyle elements are, again, essential. But by the time most people recognize the importance of blood pressure in heart health, that pressure has already begun to creep up. Thus it's not just a matter of prevention but one of vital need for a cure, for a way to get blood pressure down safely and effectively. My research has been thrilling for me, and the results I've achieved are as dramatic as those I managed for cholesterol. So it's with a great deal of delight that I guide you through what I've learned about the "secret weapons" against high blood pressure.

You're about to read a wonderful story that took decades to develop from research all over the world. It's a medical detective tale, complete with mystery and discovery. Three of the main characters won the Nobel Prize in medicine. Four plant-derived supplements are recognized for their abilities to lower blood pressure naturally. And thanks to all those efforts, you and I are the real winners in our fight against hypertension.

When we talk about heart disease, we're really talking about a disease of the arteries that supply blood to the heart muscle. A heart attack occurs when the coronary arteries fail to get enough blood to that muscle and it begins to die from lack of oxygen. A stroke happens when the carotid arteries in the neck can't provide sufficient blood and oxygen to the brain, most typically when a clot forms in a narrowed carotid artery. In discussions of cholesterol, smoking, blood pressure, and other risk factors, we tend to forget the importance of the arteries themselves.

When most people think about the arteries at all, it's in terms of plumbing. The arteries are simply pipes, conduits, for blood flow. Problems occur when those pipes get clogged, although not in the simplistic way that's commonly imagined. The plaque, as arterial blockage is properly termed, doesn't accumulate on the inner walls of the arteries the way calcium builds up on bathroom plumbing. Rather, it's a complex process that develops inside the layers of the walls of those arteries.

How and why does that blockage occur? For many years, the vast majority of researchers focused on the blockage itself, disregarding the "pipe" that was being clogged. Studies beginning in the 1950s showed a correlation between cholesterol levels and cardiovascular disease. Other risk factors, including cigarette smoking and hypertension, were also revealed. Then we learned that the principal villain in the cholesterol family is LDL and that HDL is the good guy. LDL circulates in the bloodstream and forms arterial blockage when levels become excessive. HDL does exactly the opposite, carrying cholesterol away from tissues back to the liver where it can be disposed of.

Painstaking investigations gradually described the chemical and cellular processes by which LDL penetrates the lining of the arteries and, in concert with a variety of blood cells, smooth muscle cells, and other materials, slowly but surely builds up clumps of plaque in the walls of the arteries. It was quite logical to seek ways that those processes could be interrupted to prevent or slow the blockage that would limit blood flow and that could result in a heart attack or a stroke.

Healthy Arteries, Healthy Heart and Circulation

Certainly, we still want to keep levels of LDL, triglycerides, glucose, and inflammation as low as possible. We know that by doing so we can slow, stop, and even reverse the disease process. But there's another way of looking at heart disease. Instead of looking at the blockage itself and the materials that form that blockage, scientists today are concentrating more on the artery itself.

At this point in the story, I must introduce some terms you're probably not familiar with and that you may never have heard of. It's sort of like learning the strange, unpronounceable names of characters in fantasy books such as *Lord of the Rings*.

Let's start by saying that an artery is not a solid tube like a bathroom pipe. Rather, there are three layers: the inner layer called the *intima*, the middle layer termed the *media*, and the outer layer named the *adventitia*. Finally, separating the muscular layers of the artery from the flow of blood through the open space called the *lumen*, we have a lining of flat cells termed the *endothelium*.

In the old days, people used the term *hardening of the arteries*. While we don't hear that expression much anymore, it's still an important concept. The medical term is *arteriosclerosis*, coming from the Greek words for "artery" and "hardening or stiffening," which has largely been replaced by the word *atherosclerosis*, combining the Greek words for "gruel" and "hardening." Atherosclerosis describes the disease very well, since the disease is characterized by a hardening of the artery and a deposition of plaque that has the consistency of gruel or oatmeal in the arterial walls.

Think about that for a moment. When we're young, our arteries are nice and flexible, without any blockage. As we age, the arteries stiffen and become blocked by plaque deposits, both of which limit the flow of blood. Kids can play games and sports that get their hearts beating like crazy, forcing blood through soft, elastic arteries to the muscles that need more oxygen, all without risk. But if an adult overexerts himself or herself or experiences extreme stress, the blocked and hardened arteries can't get blood through to the muscles of the heart or to the brain. And sometimes plaque ruptures, spilling its contents into the bloodstream where a clot forms. Small clots can travel through even narrowed arteries, but large clots can get stuck, stopping the blood flow. The result is a heart attack or a "brain attack"—that is, a stroke.

Here's how we tie these seemingly unrelated concepts together. Over the course of a lifetime, the endothelium, the lining of the artery, is subjected to a series of tiny injuries that cause damage. Innocently enough, the body tries to heal itself, to repair those little rips in the endothelium. It does so by bringing in blood cells, LDL, and muscle cells to form a kind of seal. Over a period of time that seal grows larger and larger and the plaque inside the walls of the artery bulges outward into the lumen, slowing the flow of blood. At the same time, as we age, our arteries stiffen and are no longer capable of stretching like rubber bands to expand and allow extra blood flow when needed. Blood pressure gradually increases, sometimes to the point of hypertension.

Recognizing that both the arterial plaque and the artery itself are involved in the disease process, scientists today approach the problem from both directions. Yet the research effort is slow, spanning the course of decades. Imagine a huge jigsaw puzzle, put together one piece at a time until the final picture emerges. Sometimes scientists believe they see the picture, only to find out years later that a missing piece of the puzzle now reveals a very different picture. The good news is that we have more of those pieces of the puzzle put together and we're getting a better look at the picture of cardiovascular disease than we've ever had before.

The Smoking Gun

In the late 1980s, researchers stumbled upon one puzzle piece in the picture of a healthy endothelium. They realized that the endothelium itself released some sort of substance that promoted *compliance*, the medical word for elasticity and flexibility, of the artery. Whatever it was, it was released, performed its action, and disappeared in a fraction of a second. Trying to identify that mysterious substance was like grabbing a handful of smoke. Even before identifying it, though, investigators began to study the manner in which it kept the artery healthy. Rather than referring to it as "it," they came up with the term *EDRF*, standing for endothelium-derived relaxation factor.

For years, articles in the medical literature detailed the activities and the functions of EDRF. Even before scientists knew what it was, they recognized the enormous importance of EDRF. Despite the difficulty of isolating and identifying something that appeared and disappeared in a nanosecond, EDRF was discovered to be a gas, nitric oxide (NO). That discovery earned three doctors the Nobel Prize in medicine in 1998.

Although EDRF/NO is relatively new in the world of pharmacology, its impact has been enormous. In just twenty-five years, more than 31,000 papers have been published with NO in the title and more than 65,000 refer to it in some way. That represents a lot of work, pieces of the jigsaw puzzle put together in laboratories, clinics, and medical centers globally!

After identification, the next step was to determine how NO was made in the endothelium. As with other bodily substances, NO manufacture involves a pathway that requires other chemical entities. The substrate, or raw material required, is an amino acid (a building block of protein), called L-arginine, henceforth in this book simply *arginine*. A special enzyme, endothelial nitric oxide synthase (eNOS), must be present for NO to be fabricated from arginine. Both of those discoveries were made in 1993, and a year earlier a different form of arginine, asymmetrical dimethyl arginine (ADMA), had been found to inhibit NO synthesis.

Blood pressure is strongly influenced by the amount of NO in the blood. In addition to relaxing the arteries and making them more compliant and able to constrict and dilate as needed, NO inhibits what doctors refer to as ACE, angiotensin converting enzyme, which raises blood pressure. Indeed, one of the commonly prescribed antihypertensive categories of drugs is that of the ACE-inhibitors. As we age, levels of NO decline and, not surprisingly, blood pressure goes up. It should be apparent to the most casual observer that if we can increase NO production, arteries will get healthier, ACE will be inhibited, and blood pressure will go down. This is my program's mode of action, the "war plan" of the secret weapons against blood pressure.

Many medical authorities in the Western world use the term *premature vascular aging* in referring to arterial stiffening as we get older, noting that some individuals' arteries stiffen earlier than others', which leads to premature heart problems. Personally I disagree with that assessment since in most populations of the world, other than in Western countries, arteries do not stiffen with age. That's because the causes of such stiffening—cigarette smoking, sedentary behavior, diabetes, elevations in cholesterol levels and blood pressure, and overweight—don't come into play.

Be that as it may, we know today that a major factor leading to arterial stiffening and subsequent hypertension is an inadequate supply of NO in the endothelium. As noted by the international hypertension authority Dr. John Cockcroft in the United Kingdom, since NO is now known to regulate, at least in part, stiffening in the arteries, therapeutic efforts to increase NO availability may prevent or reverse the problem.

Certain drugs, including the ACE inhibitors, have been shown to increase NO production. But, as we will discover shortly, there is a way to boost NO with a simple, harmless dietary supplement. There is no such thing as an NO supplement, per se, but the amino acid I'll discuss aids the body's own production of the substance.

If NO could be bottled as tablets or capsules, it would be declared a wonder drug and would make a pharmaceutical company a huge fortune. This simple little gas comprised of one molecule of nitrogen and one of oxygen performs a variety of wonders in the body. NO improves the ability of arteries to dilate, inhibits blood cells called platelets from aggregating and forming clots, limits the production of smooth muscle cells that contribute to the formation of arterial plaque, regulates the oxygenation of cells, mediates cellular defense systems, and functions as a neurotransmitter in both the central and the peripheral nervous systems.

As we age, the body produces less and less NO, especially when LDL cholesterol levels are high, when we smoke cigarettes, when we gain weight, when we live sedentary lifestyles, and when we develop type 2 diabetes and sugar levels rise in the blood. Reduced production of NO leads to arterial constriction that limits blood flow, elevates blood pressure, increases blood clot production, and results in more rapid cell death and cardiovascular disease. For reasons yet to be determined, blacks produce less NO than whites do, which may explain why the incidence of hypertension is higher in that community. And while there is an association, we don't know whether a decreased production of NO contributes to the development of type 2 diabetes or whether that form of diabetes results in less NO. Decreased NO production has also been correlated with the early development of atherosclerosis. In 2005, Russian scientists at the Scientific Sessions of the American Heart Association reported their findings that a decline in NO production parallels increases in blood pressure from mild to severe.

You don't need a Ph.D. or an M.D. degree to see why it would be nice to have more NO produced in our bodies, but it did take hundreds of men and women with those degrees and others, working in labs and medical centers internationally, to figure out ways to maintain and increase NO production. You and I owe those people a huge debt, and following the recommendations stemming from their findings will help us to lower our blood pressure levels and reduce our risk of having heart attacks and strokes.

As noted earlier, known risk factors for developing heart disease and hypertension in general, including high LDL counts, smoking, obesity, and sedentary behavior, contribute to a decreased production of NO in the endothelium. So we have more reason to get those factors under control.

I spoke of pharmaceutical companies earlier. It's no surprise that the pharmaceutical industry is hard at work developing drugs to improve NO status. One now being introduced is nebivolol, a drug in the beta-blocker family that is frequently prescribed by physicians to treat hypertension. Nebivolol is said to increase NO in the endothelium more than other beta-blockers do. But all of these drugs have side effects, as detailed in chapter 16.

It would be better if we could rev up NO production without drugs. We can do just that with four unique antioxidants taken as dietary supplements. So now we turn to the payoff in this story, with four ways to increase NO and protect our arteries while lowering blood pressure dramatically.

The Blood Pressure Cure Secret Weapon #1: Arginine

Let's start with this one because arginine is the raw material, the substrate, from which NO is made in the endothelium. To get the job done, you must have an adequate amount of eNOS, the enzyme that acts as a catalyst in the production process, and enough of the amino acid arginine. But the process can be blocked by high levels of asymmetric dimethylarginine (ADMA), a known inhibitor of NO synthesis.

What can you do to help in the process? At this time, testing for ADMA is rare and is restricted to major research centers. That's a shame, since high ADMA levels have been associated with nearly quadrupling the risk of having heart attacks and strokes by undermining the health of the endothelium, a condition known as endothelial dysfunction. On a practical level, though, you won't have access to ADMA testing. That said, you can override ADMA by increasing your blood concentrations of arginine. Sufficient arginine, in turn, leads to the production of adequate amounts of eNOS. And with enough arginine and eNOS present in the arteries, the endothelium can produce NO. We can optimize NO and lessen endothelial dysfunction, then, by supplementing with arginine. Numerous studies have demonstrated the benefits of arginine supplementation. In twelve studies from 1991 through 2005, arginine was shown to improve blood flow by improving endothelial function. Seven out of ten people showed a significant reduction in angina pain, which results from insufficient blood and oxygen reaching the heart muscle, the myocardium. Another investigation showed the benefit of arginine in improving exercise capacity. Patients suffering from congestive heart failure showed significantly improved blood flow, arterial compliance (elasticity and flexibility to allow for greater dilation), and functional status.

Men, in particular, will appreciate another benefit of arginine and the subsequent increase of NO. Cardiovascular disease affects not only coronary arteries supplying blood to the heart muscle and carotid arteries providing flow to the brain but also the arteries channeling blood into the penis to achieve an erection. As those penile arteries stiffen and become blocked with atherosclerosis, lessened blood flow leads to what is now termed *erectile dysfunction*, a polite term for male impotence. Viagra (sildenafil) is one drug in a family of agents that improve erectile dysfunction. They all share the same mode of action: increasing the production of NO to improve arterial blood flow. Viagra was first investigated as a drug for heart patients; erectile dysfunction improvement was a fortuitous side effect. Oral supplementation with arginine has demonstrated the same benefit.

Pulmonary hypertension is a very different disease from the more common systemic hypertension. It occurs in people with sickle-cell disease and sometimes in newborns. Pulmonary hypertension, it now appears, involves arginine metabolism and NO availability. Arginine supplementation has been shown to improve this disease by increasing levels of the substrate for NO production.

I have been tracking the research with arginine and NO for many years, but there has been a major stumbling block limiting the practicality of supplementing with arginine. The studies I've referred to thus far have used either intravenous administration of arginine to achieve high concentrations in the endothelium in a short period of time or extremely large oral dosages of arginine supplements. How large? Doctors have given patients doses from 5 to 15 grams daily, with most studies averaging 8 to 9 grams.

Typical arginine supplements provide 500 mg of the amino acid per capsule. That's one-half gram. To get, for example, 9 grams of arginine, one would have to swallow eighteen capsules a day, on an hourly basis for best effect. That would be both impractical and very expensive.

Oral arginine is absorbed and metabolized rapidly. Most of a given dosage would be gone in less than an hour.

In reading and hearing about the work with arginine in clinical settings, and the drawbacks of arginine supplements, I was reminded of my experiences with niacin, which is used to lower levels of LDL cholesterol and raise HDL counts. There was no doubt, going back literally decades, that niacin was wonderfully effective, but it was seldom recommended by physicians because research in the 1970s and into the 1980s indicated the need for very high dosages, which far too frequently resulted in what were termed *nuisance* side effects of flushing and gastric upset. While doctors might consider those mere nuisances, patients simply refused to take the niacin. Then in the late 1980s, about the time my cholesterol book was published, a small company developed a sustained-release formulation that drastically reduced both the dosage amount and the side effects of niacin. I describe that product, Endur-acin, in detail in my chapter on cholesterol control in this book. Could there be a sustained-release arginine?

Indeed, in 2004, Thorne Research developed the first such product, which it calls Perfusia-SR. Each capsule contains 350 mg, with directions to take three pills twice daily, in the morning and the evening. Dr. Alan L. Miller, a technical adviser at Thorne, advises patients to take the capsules in the morning with breakfast and at dinner in the evening. That adds up to just over 2 grams, far short of the 8 to 9 grams previously used. But thanks to the sustained-release formulation, arginine remains in the blood for the entire day and night, working its wonders. Thus it's not necessary to consume such large doses.

Research done at the University of Texas by Dr. Lance Gould provided dramatic evidence of arginine's potential. Dr. Gould is a recognized expert in cardiac imaging, taking pictures of the heart at work. He used a technique called a PET scan; that stands for positive emission tomography. A PET scan shows how well the heart is being "perfused," supplied with blood through the coronary arteries, and it does so in colors that portray the heart muscle getting less or more blood and oxygen. Dr. Gould took PET pictures before and after patients received Perfusia-SR. You can see the results for yourself by visiting www.thorne.com. The sustained-release arginine one-month program greatly increased blood and oxygen perfusion of the heart.

Of the twenty-nine volunteers in the study, 63 percent experienced a drop in blood pressure as well. Systolic blood pressure came down by an average of 4.1 points, and diastolic pressure was reduced by an average of 3.7 points. Those are averages across the board, whether or not the subjects had elevated blood pressure to begin with. Individuals with normal, or just slightly elevated blood pressure showed little or no benefit, but people who were borderline or hypertensive (more than 130/85) achieved a systolic reduction averaging 10.5 points with a diastolic drop of 4.9 points. Those improvements are comparable to the results achieved with prescription drugs. I expect—and hope—that we'll see much more research with sustained-release arginine in the future. This is a new frontier.

I've asked a number of physicians in private practice—real-world doctors, not those in university research centers—to experiment a bit with newly diagnosed hypertensive patients. The results have been terrific. One doctor, a family physician in Florida, was so amazed that he called with something close to disbelief. The patient was a forty-year-old man with a blood pressure of 155/102 on average. After taking SR arginine for one month, that pressure was down to 120/73. It appears that the higher the blood pressure to begin with, the better the results will be.

But here's the sad story behind the reason why I selected that particular patient to tell you about. After hearing the results, I said to Dr. Walsh in Florida, "Of course, you gave him the information for reordering the arginine so he can maintain those good results." Sadly, that was not the case. It turned out that it was less expensive for the man to get a prescription drug through his insurance plan than for him to buy the side effect–free supplement, and the patient elected to take the drug. The moral of this story is that ultimately it will be your decision whether to do nothing and remain at risk, to pay out of pocket for a harmless and very helpful dietary supplement, or to take a prescription drug.

I must, however, disclose one study that showed a risk in taking supplemental arginine. Researchers at Johns Hopkins Medical Institutions in Baltimore, Maryland, worked with 153 patients, each of whom had suffered a heart attack just three to twenty-one days before being given either 9 grams (3 grams three times daily) of arginine or a placebo for six months. Of those patients, seventy-seven were older than sixty years of age. During that period, there were twelve cardiovascular events (heart attacks, deaths, and hospitalizations for heart failure) in the arginine group and seven in the placebo group. There were six deaths in the arginine group, and none in the placebo group.

How could that have happened? Well, one must look beyond the newspaper headlines. The subjects were seriously ill following those heart attacks. One died from a rupture in the heart muscle; this would certainly not be associated with arginine in any way. Two died from sepsis, severe infections. Certainly, this will stimulate additional research. But in the meantime I don't feel that one isolated study should negate the positive findings of all the other studies. I am reminded of a lone journal article that got a lot of attention in its day back in the 1990s, reporting that there was no cholesterol improvement in people taking phytosterols, the plant sterols that are known to lower levels by 10 percent on average. That article still makes researchers scratch their collective heads, but prior and subsequent findings put it in the category of fluke. I think the same will be true for this L-arginine study. Personally, I still take the sustained-release L-arginine.

In addition to blood pressure–lowering benefits, arginine, especially in the sustained-release formulation that keeps a more-or-less constant level in the bloodstream, promotes the health of the endothelium. That's been well established in a large number of clinical studies. Remember that arginine is the body's *only* substrate—raw material, as it were—for NO production. Without sufficient supplies in the body, we cannot make enough NO for optimal arterial health.

For reasons not totally understood yet—and I'm certain that as time goes on, we'll have more and more knowledge, owing to the incredible importance of this new field of heart health—arginine works best for people who have blood pressure levels of more than 130/80. Individuals in the lower categories termed prehypertensive, could, inexplicably, take arginine without seeing an improvement while people with much higher numbers, such as Dr. Walsh's patient, will experience complete normalization.

For more information on Perfusia-SR, visit www.perfusia .com (for sales information) and www.thorne.com (for additional research details, including before and after PET scan images).

While Thorne was the first company to develop a sustained-release arginine capsule, another company with an outstanding performance record and an international reputation in sustained-release formulations has perfected a 350 mg tablet that delivers even more predictable and consistent blood levels of arginine. The Endurance Products Company of Tigard, Oregon, now markets this product as EP L-Arginine SR. Having developed a unique system of sustained-release delivery of other supplements, including niacin, vitamin C, and others, Endurance Products can be completely trusted that its arginine will provide maximum benefit. Its system of sustained release of arginine is actually superior to that of Perfusia-SR. Another major difference is that it is significantly cheaper than Thorne's product and there is no charge for shipping. Call Endurance Products Company at (800) 483-2532 for an order form or visit www.endur.com.

If you live outside the United States, place orders for the Endurance sustained-release arginine tablets at www.endur.com; click on Customer Service, International Orders. In the United States, order directly from Endurance products at www.endur.com.

My personal cardiologist, Steven Burstein, M.D., at Good Samaritan Hospital in Los Angeles, who is also associate professor of medicine at UCLA Medical School, agreed to test the Endurance sustained-release arginine. He did so with several patients who were diagnosed as having prehypertension, with systolic blood pressure between 120 and 139. He found that the arginine, taken as directed—three tablets in the morning and three in the evening—lowered systolic blood pressure by nearly 10 points in most individuals, and never less than 5 points.

That's dramatic, especially in view of the current hypertension management guidelines used by physicians that point out that a 5-point reduction in systolic blood pressure can reduce mortality substantially and reduce the risk of stroke by 14 percent and the incidence of coronary heart disease by 9 percent.

I hereby disclose that I have absolutely no financial interest in any of the products or the companies I have discussed in this chapter. I receive no compensation of any kind from the purchase of any or all of the secret weapons.

The good news is that there are more weapons in our blood pressure–lowering armamentarium. The next one we'll consider has been shown to do a wonderful job of dealing with those lower levels of blood pressure elevation.

The Blood Pressure Cure Secret Weapon #2: Grape Seed Extract

Since ancient times, grapes have been held in high regard for promoting health. You can find references to recommendations for increased grape eating by physicians, including by Hippocrates, virtually everywhere in the world where grapes have been grown. Grapes and their vines have decorated everything from clothing to vases throughout history. John Harvey Kellogg, M.D., the man who began the Kellogg cereal empire, prescribed ten to fourteen pounds (yes, pounds, not grams or even ounces) of grapes daily as a remedy for high blood pressure. No, don't worry, I'm not going to suggest that you do that! Fortunately, we've learned a lot since those days, and the solution is a lot more practical.

While you may never have heard of Dr. Kellogg's grape obsession, you certainly know about what's called the "French paradox." Why does France have a remarkably low rate of heart disease and deaths from this disease despite having a diet that's rich in the foods most health authorities tell us to cut way back on? Could it be the red wine that the French wash those foods down with?

Actually, subsequent studies—and there have been hundreds of them—have determined that the main benefit of regular wine consumption comes from the alcohol, which raises levels of the protective HDL cholesterol. Along those lines, beer, spirits, or whatever might be your drink of choice will do the same thing. But there is something very special about that red wine, which gets its color from having the grape skins left in the vats during the fermentation process. White wine lacks the red color because the skins are removed. We've learned that the red color comes from a special class of plant substances called polyphenols, powerful agents that came under scientific scrutiny only in the mid-1900s. There are literally thousands of those polyphenols in fruits, vegetables, and all plants and plant-derived foods. Why did it take science so long to recognize the value of these substances? Probably the biggest reason research got a slow start was and still is the enormous diversity and complexity of their chemical structures.

Relax, there's no reason for you to learn the intricate nuances of the wonderful world of polyphenols. Suffice it to say that current data very strongly support a combination of polyphenols in their roles in the prevention and cure of cardiovascular diseases, cancers, diabetes, and degenerative nerve diseases. Although polyphenols have been under the scientific microscope for just over a decade, the wealth of knowledge built up thus far is fantastic, and new information is literally being added weekly to the scientific and medical literature in journals all over the world. The internationally prestigious *American Journal of Clinical Nutrition* included an entire 120-page, 17-article supplement, "Dietary Polyphenols and Health," along with its January 2005 issue.

Much of the polyphenol research has concentrated on cardio-vascular disease, and today it is well established that polyphenols, consumed as foods or supplements, improve health status and reduce cardiovascular risk. Much of that body of investigation has involved laboratory animals, but we now have enough human clin-ical studies to prove their benefits for us as well as for mice and rats. One such study showed how rats given grape seed extract (GSE) following induced heart attacks suffered far less damage. My own interest in GSE, a particularly rich source of certain polyphenols, began in 2003 when I read that when it was fed to mice, their blood pressure levels came down appreciably. I wrote about that study in my newsletter and began adding GSE to my own supplement regi-men. To my delight, I saw a very nice improvement, but more about blood pressure control in just a bit.

Any reading about polyphenols in the medical journals inevitably leads us back to the health of the endothelium and the role of nitric oxide (NO). Truly, that's where the action is, with good reason, since NO has vital abilities to help arterial dilation, prevent inflammation, limit the formation of blood clots, and, in general, pro-mote arterial health. In that special *AJCN* supplement, one of the most prominently discussed sources of polyphenols was GSE. That's because GSE has one of the highest concentrations of those potent substances. Just a little bit goes a long way.

To get the natural antioxidant and artery-protecting benefits of just one 200 mg grape seed extract tablet or capsule, you would have to drink 4 ounces of red wine or 6 ounces of red grape juice or eat a serving of various fruits. To think that for centuries, grape seeds were discarded as waste during the production of wine!

When postmenopausal women took a daily dose of 100 mg to 500 mg of GSE, they lowered their systolic pressure by 20 points. Interestingly, the salt content of those women's diets was particularly high. The better recommendation, I think, would be to ease up on the salt while taking grape seed extract tablets or capsules.

Much of the investigation into the benefits of GSE has been

done at the University of California at Davis by the professor of cardiovascular medicine C. Tissa Kappagoda. At the Experimental Biology Conference in San Diego in April 2003, he and his associates presented the findings of three such studies. Dr. Kappagoda described GSE as "a powerful antioxidant" that has a significant effect on atherosclerosis by preventing cholesterol from accumulating in the arteries.

In two of the studies, the UC Davis team gave GSE along with a high-fat diet to one group of guinea pigs. The other guinea pigs did not receive GSE. After twelve weeks, the cholesterol accumulation in the animals' arteries was significantly lower in the group receiving GSE. A third study the team described at that meeting showed that GSE inhibited the atherosclerotic effects of the highly saturated fat in coconut oil.

But you and I are neither rats nor mice nor guinea pigs. The good news is that research has shown benefits for humans as well. One study showed how GSE "supercharged" vitamins E and C in humans to provide greater antioxidant capabilities than the vitamins alone had. A British project revealed how the polythenols of GSE help to restore endothelial function by inhibiting a substance called endothelin-1. Most recently, truly exciting breakthroughs have come in the use of GSE to lower blood pressure in two types of patients.

The first investigation, also done by the UC Davis team, involved twenty-four male and female patients diagnosed with what is termed *metabolic syndrome*, categorized by overweight, insulin resistance and resultantly higher levels of the blood sugar glucose, low counts of the protective HDL cholesterol along with high concentrations of triglycerides, and elevated blood pressure. The patients were divided into three groups of eight. The first group got a placebo, the second was given 150 mg of a specially formulated GSE, and the third took 300 mg of GSE. Each patient took a single dose once a day. Participants' blood pressure readings were automatically measured and recorded twelve hours at the beginning and end of the one-month study.

While there was no blood pressure change in the placebo group, Dr. Kappagoda first announced at the March 26, 2006, meeting of the American Chemical Society, that participants in the other two groups achieved an equal degree of blood pressure reduction, averaging 12 mm Hg systolic and 8 mm Hg diastolic. People taking the 300 mg dosage also reduced their serum LDL cholesterol. The higher the LDL to begin with, the better the improvement.

Dr. Kappagoda is now concluding a second investigation of the remarkable capabilities of MegaNatural-BP with men and women diagnosed with prehypertension, whose systolic levels are from 120 to 139 and diastolic levels are from 80 to 89. Prehypertension is estimated to affect 31 percent of the entire U.S. population, 39 percent of men and 23 percent of women. Contrary to popular belief, those elevated blood pressure levels now termed prehypertension affect more than 37 percent of African Americans, 32.2 percent of whites, and 30.9 percent of Hispanics between 20 and 39 years of age—not just middle-aged and older people.

Subjects in the UC Davis prehypertension study had a baseline systolic pressure averaging 134.1 and a diastolic reading of 79.1. Thirty participants completed the study. As Dr. Kappagoda reported in April 2007 at the meeting of the Federation of American Societies for Experimental Biology, blood pressures were measured automatically at the start, midpoint, and end of the eight-week study. No difference was noted in the blood pressures of the placebo group, but those in the group receiving 300 mg of Mega-Natural-BP daily had average reductions down to 125.8 systolic and 73.4 diastolic. That is a decrease of about 8 points systolic and 6 points diastolic. Such reductions can significantly reduce the risk of heart attack and stroke.

While GSE has been shown to have a blood pressure–lowering effect in other, earlier studies, it was pleasantly surprising to see such impressive improvements with rather low GSE dosages. Based on previous animal studies, which usually correlate pretty closely on a milligram-dosage-per-kilogram-or-pound-of-weight basis to humans, one would have predicted the need for much higher dosages to achieve that sort of blood pressure lowering.

The reason is a specially formulated GSE that concentrates a specific isolate that has the greatest blood pressure–lowering potency. It is made by the Polyphenolics company and sold as

MegaNatural-BP grape seed extract under a variety of brands, as well as directly from the company. This is the formulation of GSE used in the Kappagoda clinical studies. While one might expect blood pressure lowering from ordinary GSE, no detailed human studies have been done to establish necessary dosages, although they would be significantly higher than those needed with the MegaNatural-BP. At least one study has shown that ordinary GSE does not have a blood pressure–lowering effect.

Visit www.polyphenolics.com to find MegaNatural-BP grape seed extract. What about drinking grape juice? It's a wonderful source of those polyphenols, and I strongly recommend it. You'll find a number of ways of using grape juice concentrate in the recipe section at the end of the book. But to get a major benefit, you'd have to drink a lot of grape juice every day. In another study reported at the 2003 meeting of the Federation of American Societies for Experimental Biology, men who drank 12 ounces of red grape juice daily for twelve weeks had a drop in systolic blood pressure from 142.7 to 137.0, while diastolic pressure went down from 87.9 to 82.1. That's nice, but I wonder how practical it would be in real life.

The Blood Pressure Cure Secret Weapon #3: Tomato Extract

Even people who have been taking blood pressure–lowering drugs will benefit from this natural choice. And individuals who are determined to get their blood pressure down without drugs will benefit enormously. Tomato extract, which is rich in the antioxidant polyphenols lycopene, phytoene, and phytofluene, has been shown to reduce blood pressure for treated but not completely controlled hypertensive individuals, as well as for never-treated men and women in the category of prehypertension. Two studies have been done at the University of the Negev in Beer Sheva, Israel, by Dr. Esther Paran and her colleagues.

Published in the *American Heart Journal*, the first study involved thirty-one men and women who had not taken antihypertensive drugs but had been diagnosed as having higher than normal blood pressure. This was a placebo-controlled study in which the patients were given a single daily dose of a commonly available tomato extract product, Lyc-O-Mato, containing 15 mg of lycopene, 1 mg of phytofluene, 1 mg of phytoene, and the antioxidants beta-carotene and vitamin E. No other supplements were allowed.

Participants in the study included adults thirty to seventy years of age whose blood pressures were between 140 and 159 mm Hg systolic and 90 and 99 mm Hg diastolic. For the first four weeks, they took a placebo and their blood pressures were monitored and recorded. Then they took the Lyc-O-Mato tomato extract for eight weeks, after which they returned to another month of placebo capsules. During the treatment period, average systolic blood pressure readings fell from an average of 144 to 134 while average diastolic declines went from 87.4 to 83.4. That drop of 10 points systolic and 4 points diastolic is about as much as any single antihypertensive drug can achieve. A significant improvement was noted after the first six weeks of taking the extract and it continued through the entire eight-week test period. No improvements occurred during the placebo stages, with blood pressure returning to pretreatment levels when the placebo replaced the extract. There were no changes in weight or physical activity during the study. The only factor operating in the blood pressure improvement was the tomato extract.

The aim of the second Israeli study with tomato extract was to evaluate the potential change in systolic and diastolic blood pressure in treated but uncontrolled hypertensive patients after an eight-week treatment period. Dr. Paran and her colleagues also studied changes in nitric oxide during treatment. This was the gold standard of medical research: a randomized, double-blind, crossover, placebo-controlled study.

There were fifty-four subjects whose blood pressures remained elevated despite the use of antihypertensive drugs. Often two or three different drugs are required to completely control hypertension, but such combinations frequently lead to side effects that commonly limit patients' compliance with doctors' prescriptions. Dr. Paran hoped that the tomato extract would offer an alternative to adding another drug or two.

Patients were from thirty to seventy years of age and did not have other disease problems. After a routine baseline evaluation to determine weight, blood pressure, and blood values, including cholesterol, study participants entered two double-blind, cross-over treatment periods of six weeks each, with either daily tomato extract (Lyc-O-Mato) or a placebo. Neither the doctors nor the patients knew who was taking which, and following the first phase, the groups were "crossed over" to give people previously on the placebo the tomato extract and vice versa.

During the study, both blood pressure readings and levels of the metabolite of nitric oxide, nitrate, were measured and recorded. NO levels were significantly increased, and blood pressure averages dropped by 8 to 11 mm Hg systolic and 3 to 5 mm Hg diastolic. That's about what doctors would hope for in adding a second antihypertensive prescription drug.

Previous research with the DASH study (Dietary Approaches to Stopping Hypertension) showed that increasing fruits, vegetables, and whole grains in the diet for eight weeks could lower blood pressure, with average reductions of 2.8 points systolic and 1.1 points diastolic. Compare those numbers with the improvements from using tomato extract! Could one simply choose to increase tomato consumption? Perhaps, but one Lyc-O-Mato capsule is the equivalent of eating *four* tomatoes daily, and those tomatoes would have to be cooked to release the lycopene for best bioavailability. Moreover, lycopene itself, isolated from other polyphenols in Lyc-O-Mato tomato extract, does *not* have a blood pressure–lowering effect.

No doubt, there will be more research data with lycopene and tomato extract in the future. It may be, for example, that there will be a dose-dependent effect. That is to say, increasing the dosage may yield even better results. As one example of how, in this case, more may be better, research has shown that a dosage of 60 mg of lycopene daily reduced LDL cholesterol by 14 percent. Dr. Paran pointed out to me via e-mail that people with higher blood pressure levels to begin with showed the most significant improvements. Could boosting the dosage also help to bring your blood pressure down lower? Or might you be able to achieve a lower blood pressure by combining lycopene tomato extract with one of the other "secret weapons" of this chapter? As one anatomy professor once taught me, we're all as different on the inside as we are on the outside. It would certainly be worth your while to experiment a bit. You have nothing to lose, since all these potent weapons have no potential for harm, and everything to gain.

Lyc-O-Mato is widely available in stores and on the Internet. Check your local pharmacy or health food store. Or, for additional information, visit www.lycored.com or www.lycopene.com.

The Blood Pressure Cure Secret Weapon #4: Pycnogenol

Pycnogenol has a wonderful tale of discovery all its own, going back literally centuries to the time of the early exploration of North America. During Jacques Cartier's expeditions in Canada, searching for a northwest passage to China, he found himself trapped in the frozen Hudson Bay in the winter of 1535. Having depleted their supplies of fresh food, his men began developing scurvy. Twenty-five had already died and fifty more were seriously ill when Cartier was offered help from Chief Domagaia, who prepared a tea made from pine needles and bark that was drunk several times a day by the ailing men. Within one to two weeks, the symptoms of scurvy subsided and the men recovered fully.

As a side note, remember that the most frequently used drug, aspirin, was discovered by Native Americans who brewed the bark of the willow tree to treat aches and pains. Of course, they didn't realize that the brown tea they shared with early settlers contained what scientists came to identify as acetylsalicylic acid, more commonly known as aspirin. It was only within recent decades that medical researchers have determined just how aspirin works its anti-inflammatory and painkilling wonders by altering hormonelike substances called prostaglandins.

Going back to Pycnogenol and how it helped Cartier's men fight scurvy, it took centuries to learn that the pine needles provided a small amount of vitamin C and the bark yielded vitamin C–supercharging bioflavonoids, members of the polyphenol family of plant-derived substances. In fact, it was only in 1984 that scientists identified and quantified the compounds in Pycnogenol.

Today Pycnogenol is obtained exclusively from a tree called the French maritime pine that grows in a 4,000-square-mile area of forest along the Bay of Biscay, bordered by the Atlantic Ocean, between the wine-producing district of Bordeaux to the north and the Pyrenees Mountains to the south. It is sold under a number of brand names throughout the world and has earned a pedigree of benefits that is truly remarkable, acting as an extremely potent antioxidant and stimulating the enzyme eNOS (endothelial nitric oxide synthase) to produce nitric oxide (NO) in the arterial linings from arginine. Ah, so now I'll bet you've already made the connection and discovered the reason why arginine and Pycnogenol are two of my secret weapons, working hand in hand with each other in the fight against high blood pressure!

Let's tie things together a little more tightly. Remember my explanation of how the ACE inhibitor drugs that are prescribed for hypertension will work to reduce angiotensin converting enzyme? In 1996, German and Hungarian researchers, working in collaboration, found that Pycnogenol has a dose-dependent ability to block ACE from raising blood pressure. People with normal blood pressure wouldn't be affected at all, but individuals with elevated blood pressure owing to excessive levels of ACE will achieve blood pressure lowering. Antihypertensive drugs also increase levels of NO in the endothelium, relaxing the arteries for better dilation and constriction, and thereby lowering blood pressure. Again, Pycnogenol provides that benefit. Between the two modes of action, Pycnogenol has been proved safe and effective in human clinical trials. Two of the Pycnogenol studies are particularly worth noting and demonstrate its value.

In 2001, investigators at the University of Arizona at Tucson did a "gold standard" study of Pycnogenol and blood pressure. This was a randomized, double-blind, placebo-controlled, prospective, sixteen-week trial to see how well this potent antioxidant would work in modifying blood pressure in mildly hypertensive patients. Again, that's really important since so much emphasis today is being focused on numbers just a bit higher than normal, with the recognition that those numbers are forecasts of future hypertension.

In this gold standard investigation, the patients were selected at random. It was double-blind, meaning that neither doctor nor patient knew what was given, whether the active agent or a placebo sugar pill. Prospective means that it took a look forward, rather than relying on reports of what had been done by the patients in the past. And it was long enough in duration to see real effects.

Eleven men and women received either 200 mg per day of Pycnogenol or the placebo. Their blood pressure levels ranged from 140 to 159 systolic and 90 to 99 diastolic. After eight weeks, people getting the Pycnogenol were switched to the placebo and vice versa. The results were statistically significant. Average improvements dropped the systolic pressure to 133 in subjects taking Pycnogenol. The higher the blood pressure to begin with, the greater the improvement.

A second investigation, published in 2004, looked into whether Pycnogenol could be used to reduce the amount of an antihypertensive drug that people needed to take. The fifty-eight male and female patients, averaging fifty-seven years of age, in the study had been placed on 20 mg of nifedipine, a drug in the class of calcium antagonists. Over a period of twelve weeks, their blood pressure was monitored and recorded regularly, and the subjects received either a placebo or 100 mg per day of Pycnogenol. Depending on blood pressure readings every two weeks, the nifedipine dosages were adjusted to maintain lowered levels of pressure.

Most patients at the end of the twelve-week study had normal blood pressure readings and were able to cut the dosages of their drug literally in half, from 20 mg per day to just 10 mg per day, by supplementing it with 100 mg per day of Pycnogenol.

Now, here's the problem I have as a medical journalist who is also trained in medical physiology and research. I keep asking questions that have no answers because the particular study wasn't structured to resolve those questions. For example, what would have happened if the Pycnogenol dosage was increased to 200 mg per day, as was the case in the University of Arizona research? Would one see a dose-dependent response? Could those patients have been completely weaned off their prescription medications? Would the results have been even stronger if the subjects had also been instructed to decrease alcohol consumption, to get more physical activity, to practice stress management, to lose weight, and to incorporate other supplements such as arginine? Each of those questions, researchers quickly explain, introduces a variable. "Teasing" out the effects of one thing from another becomes extremely time consuming and expensive.

Thanks to the experience of one of my readers, I know that generic "pine bark extract" may not produce the blood pressure–lowering effects of Pycnogenol. That particular reader, by the way, is an M.D. involved in research at a major pharmaceutical company. He's been following my cholesterol program for many years, and started on the blood pressure program after reading about it in my publication, *The Diet-Heart Newsletter*.

That physician added supplements in steps, finally reaching his desired blood pressure goal after adding Pycnogenol. But then, to save a little money, he switched to a generic pine bark extract. Whoops! His blood pressure started coming back up. When he returned to Pycnogenol, it went right down again. Bingo. Sometimes trying to save a few dollars can be a waste of money! Use the real thing.

Pycnogenol is widely available worldwide. Shop for it on the Internet or at your local pharmacy or health food store. You can find more information at www.pycnogenol.com.

At this point let me reiterate: research with the polyphenols has only been going on since the mid-1990s. We're at the frontiers of a brave new world of alternative approaches to health maintenance in general and blood pressure control in particular. When I began to write and speak about oat bran and niacin back in the mid-1980s, we were in the same boat. Since that time, both of those approaches have been "cast in bronze" as clinically proven ways to lower cholesterol. There's no doubt in my mind that in the coming years, the use of arginine and the various polyphenolic agents, including grape seed extract, lycopene from tomato extract, and Pycnogenol, will be mainstream.

Availability of all the secret weapons will increase over time. While combination products may include one or another of these secret weapons, probably the best and most economical products will provide only one ingredient, such as Pycnogenol or

MegaNatural-BP grape seed extract. The best way to find them is through one of the Web sites I've provided.

We're all different. We all respond differently to approaches and interventions. Just think about sodium. Some people are sensitive, some are supersensitive, and others are not sensitive at all. When it comes to getting blood pressure readings to optimal levels, one size does not fit all. This book provides a foundation program that everyone should follow: get to your optimal healthy weight, increase your physical activity, definitely quit the cigarettes, manage your stress as best you can, lower your blood sugar levels if you're diabetic or borderline, and improve your diet by eating far more fruits, vegetables, and whole grains while balancing your electrolytes in terms of less sodium and more calcium, magnesium, and potassium. Heck, even if you have perfect blood pressure, you and I and everyone else should follow that lifestyle to improve our health in general.

Then do some personal experimentation. Start with arginine supplementation and perhaps one of the other secret weapons. See how you do after a month or two. If you need a bit more horsepower, add another one of the other agents. Or, if you're like me and want the best of all worlds, you can do exactly the opposite by starting with *all* of the secret weapons along with the lifestyle modifications. Perhaps you'd prefer to combine two of the agents. Again, see how well you do. Eventually, as you learn what works best for you, you can add or subtract one or another agent. With one of those inexpensive home monitoring devices, it's really easy to test yourself without going to the doctor's office as you would have to do when your goal is cholesterol control—there's no way you can test your cholesterol levels at home.

In August 2006, I did a radio interview with a man who told me following the show that his own blood pressure remained elevated at 145/93 despite taking a prescription drug. His doctor wanted to add a second drug, and the radio host was worried about side effects. Respecting his privacy, I will not reveal his name or the radio station.

I had brought bottles of two supplements, the Endurance sustained-release arginine and the MegaNatural-BP grape seed extract, for show-and-tell purposes during such interviews and presentations and had some extras. I offered the man the two bottles and gave him my e-mail address, asking him to let me know how things worked out for him.

Well, I grinned from ear to ear just a few days later when my publicist told me that the man had called to say that his blood pressure had already come down. In fact, he wanted to do a follow-up interview. By the time I spoke with him, eight days after he started to take the supplements, his blood pressure was down to 128/82. And he hadn't even begun to follow the other simple steps in my program to get those numbers down even further.

Can everyone expect improvements in blood pressure? Yes. Will there be such dramatically rapid reductions? I really don't know. Probably it will take at least a few weeks for most men and women to gear up in following the program, including taking the supplements I discuss in this chapter. I have gotten a lot of feedback from the readers of my quarterly publication, *The Diet-Heart Newsletter*, that their blood pressure levels have fallen in virtually every case. Sometimes the reductions have been very satisfying and sometimes they've been absolutely spectacular. This stuff really works!

One thing is absolutely and positively true. If you follow the recommendations I've detailed in this book, you're definitely going to feel better, sleep better, enjoy life more, and see your blood pressure come down. That should bring a smile to your face! And with that happy thought, I'll end this chapter with a sweet—quite literally sweet—way to further improve your blood pressure.

The Blood Pressure Cure Secret Weapon #5: Cocoa

I love the scene in the Woody Allen film *Sleeper* in which a physician in the distant future makes the observation that "In ancient times, people believed that hot fudge sundaes were bad for health. Can you imagine?" Well, I'm not quite ready to advocate those sundaes to promote a healthy heart, but the cocoa that goes into the fudge? Yup, it's really good for you, your heart, and your blood pressure. Lurking in the dusty medical libraries are about 150 articles published between 1996 and 2005, all extolling the benefits of chocolate and cocoa. How sweet is that?

One such study came from the University of L'Aquila in Italy where researchers have been busily looking into the cardiovascular benefits of the flavonols, a type of polyphenol, that are found in cocoa products. Dr. Claudio Ferri and his colleagues, in collaboration with investigators at Tufts University in Boston, learned that flavonol-rich dark chocolate reduces blood pressure during both the day and the night in patients with hypertension.

Not surprisingly, much of the research on cocoa has been done in the Netherlands, a country famous for its hot cocoa. A study of elderly Dutch men indicates that eating or drinking cocoa is associated with lower blood pressure and reduced mortality. Interestingly, the reduction in the death rate was *not* associated with lower blood pressure. The researchers speculate that cocoa's rich content of bioflavonols, which are potent antioxidants, may be responsible for that very desirable benefit.

Similar flavonols abound in fruits, vegetables, red wine, and green tea, but chocolate products have a higher total flavonol content on a per weight basis. Please pay close attention to that. It means that a 3½-ounce dark chocolate bar has more of those polyphenols than 3½ ounces of, say, a serving of fruit. But you're not going to substitute five or more chocolate bars for the recommended five or more servings of fruits and vegetables! As I'll show you, though, you can get all the goodness of chocolate and cocoa without the fat and the calories.

Another nice thing about the flavonols in cocoa is that they're absorbed very rapidly into the bloodstream. That might well explain why sipping a nice warm cup of cocoa before bedtime can quickly relax you for a good night's sleep.

Dr. Ferri's group has reported that dark chocolate, but not white chocolate, reduces blood pressure in healthy subjects they worked with. Then the Willy Wonka doctors wondered whether dark chocolate could actually lower blood pressure in people with hypertension. They recruited twenty patients who had never been treated for their elevated blood pressure, which was from 140 to 159 systolic and 90 to 99 diastolic, and fifteen similar individuals who had normal blood pressure readings. All of the subjects avoided red wine and green tea during the study period.

Each participant received either 100 grams per day of dark chocolate, estimated to contain 88 mg of flavonols, or 90 grams of white chocolate, devoid of flavonols, for fifteen days. Then the groups switched the types of chocolate. The results were, to say the least, impressive. Systolic blood pressure fell by 11.9 points and diastolic blood pressure came down by 8.5 points for people who ate the dark chocolate, while individuals who consumed the white chocolate showed no difference. Folks, that's a *huge* improvement, comparable to what you might get from a prescription drug. The blood pressure reductions persisted through both day and night. And as a special bonus, LDL cholesterol counts tumbled down by 10 percent. The chocolate used in the study was only the dark variety, neither white nor milk chocolate, and it was specially prepared to contain a very high level of the cocoa flavonols. White and milk chocolates have either little or none of the beneficial flavonols.

How does cocoa spin its magic spells on blood pressure? Once again, it comes down to improved levels of NO in the blood, relaxing the arteries and making them more compliant. In an editorial accompanying the article published in *Hypertension*, it was suggested that the mode of action might involve the inhibition of ACE, once again like those antihypertensive ACE-inhibitor drugs. Let's see: would I rather enjoy some cocoa or take a prescription drug? Hmm. At this very moment as I sit at my computer, I'm sipping a morning cup of coffee heavily laced with ultra-rich cocoa. More about that a bit later, but first let's review some of the research.

Although the Aztec Indians of Mexico and Central America "invented" cocoa, which was reserved for royalty, when one thinks of cocoa, Holland comes to mind. That's where much of the world's finest cocoa comes from, and cafes and restaurants in the Netherlands offer hot cocoa as a matter of course. So it's fitting that a fascinating investigation done by the National Institute for Public Health and the Environment in that country followed 470 Dutch men over a fifteen-year period. The volunteers were between the ages of sixty-five and eighty-four and were medically examined and interviewed about their diets every five years.

Over the course of the study, 314 men died, with 152 of those deaths from cardiovascular disease. Scientists determined that men who had consumed on average 4 grams of cocoa per day, about what you'd get in a few squares of dark chocolate, had significantly lower blood pressure than those who did not. But here's the real winner: they were also half as likely as the others to die from cardiovascular disease. And men with a really high cocoa consumption were less likely to die from *any* cause. No wonder those Aztec chiefs kept it to themselves!

Now back to examining some of the delicious research findings. An international team of investigators from the United States and Germany further determined that the particular flavonol in cocoa is called epicatechin, not that this tidbit of information is of particular value other than to chemists reading this book. What *is* of value is their finding that a flavonol-rich cocoa drink increased vasodilation of arteries, increased NO production, and boosted microcirculation. All those things contribute to lowering blood pressure.

Although the Aztec Indians are long gone from Mexico and Central America, other indigenous peoples have perpetuated the delicious habit of drinking cocoa. Many of the Kuna Indians on Panama's offshore islands routinely slurp three to four cups of cocoa daily. It's pretty important to note that blood pressure barely rises as these people age and that cardiovascular disease in general is rare. Maybe it's a matter of fortuitous genetics? When the Kunas move to the mainland, they lose their cocoa-drinking habits and both blood pressure and the incidence of heart disease increase. When scientists examined the island-dwelling Kunas and the mainlanders, they found that islanders have six times higher levels of the flavonol epicatechin and double the amount of NO in their blood as do the mainlanders. Cocoa powder and cocoa extracts have been shown to have higher antioxidant capacity than many other flavonol-rich foods, including both green and black teas, red wine, garlic, blueberries, and strawberries, although we should include plenty of those foods in our diets as well. Man cannot live by cocoa alone, but it's a pretty good start!

I've advocated a lot of heart-healthy foods over the decades that I've been a heart-health warrior. But not everyone is as crazy about fish as I am. Many people find oat bran pretty boring, and it takes a lot of persuasion to get folks to really boost their fruit and vegetable consumption. Then we come to cocoa.

Who doesn't like or even love chocolate and cocoa? The Aztecs were correct when they thought of cocoa as a gift of the gods. But they didn't munch on chocolate candy bars all day. They drank their cocoa, and that's what I'd like to suggest that you do as well.

Much of the research on chocolate and cocoa has been sponsored by the Mars candy company. That company has two things in mind. First, it would like to boost its sales across the board, and it has introduced specially formulated dark chocolate bars branded as CocoaVia. But please don't think of those confections as health food. To get a beneficial dose of flavonols, you'd need to munch two bars daily. That will add about 200 calories a day, which, if not off-set by increased physical activity or a decreased intake of other foods, would lead to a weight gain of 20 pounds in the first year! Those bars would also provide 36 percent of the maximum amount of saturated fat in a heart-healthy diet. Not a good idea. Read the ingredients listings of those candy bars and others and you'll see what I mean. Be prepared for an onslaught of advertising and pro-motion for the dozens of "healthy" chocolate bars launched world-wide in 2006. The Mars company's second motivation for funding research is the desire to isolate and package the active flavonols to be sold either as an over-the-counter supplement or a prescription antihypertensive drug. To think that you can get something that powerful and good for your heart, today, not some time in the dis-tant future, in a chocolate bar or a cup of cocoa.

On the other hand, savoring a couple of squares of a dark, rich chocolate bar now and then wouldn't be too bad an idea. If noth-ing else, doing so might teach you how to take a tiny bite at a time and allow it to melt on your tongue, fully enjoying the indulgent moment. But doing so should be a treat, not a daily habit. As time goes on, I'm noticing an increase in chocolate confections that tout their concentrations of cocoa, and that's a good thing, indeed. You'll find that even one little square can be remarkably satisfying.

Conversely, there's no need to limit your potential enjoyment of cocoa in many ways. I mentioned that as I've been writing this section, I've been sipping a cup of coffee laced with dark, rich cocoa.

Nothing could be simpler. Just put a heaping tablespoon (yielding about 5 grams or more of pure cocoa) or two (or three for a really intense flavor) into a cup or a mug and pour in the hot coffee. Sweeten it with either sugar or an artificial sweetener to taste. Perhaps splash in a dollop of milk. Enjoy! If you find that you like this a lot, as I do, you can even add the cocoa powder to the ground coffee beans as you make your pot in the morning or any time of the day.

At the end of a long, often stressful day of work, I love to prepare a steaming cup of hot cocoa to sip while reading a book or watching a bit of TV before bed. Just preparing it starts the process of relaxation, I guess because I know what's in store for me. This doesn't take culinary genius. Put out one of your favorite mugs. Spoon in a heaping tablespoon (or two or three tablespoons) of dark cocoa and some sweetener (you'll definitely need to sweeten it, since pure cocoa is actually on the bitter side). While doing that, you'll have some nonfat or low-fat milk warming on the stove or in the microwave. Pure the steaming milk over the cocoa and the sweetener, stir, and bring the mug to your nose as you would a fine glass of wine. Sit, sip, relax, and mellow out. You and I both deserve a nice reward at the end of a long day, and this treat will actually lower your blood pressure when enjoyed regularly.

For variety, try using some orange marmalade, raspberry or strawberry preserves, or even a tablespoon of frozen red or purple grape juice concentrate in place of sugar or other sweeteners. Combining the flavors of fruit with cocoa just can't be beat!

There are many other ways to enjoy cocoa as well. Here's a cooling suggestion for a hot summer's day. Put a dollop of cocoa powder, a fairly ripe banana, a tablespoon of honey, and a large glass of milk into a blender to swirl into a delicious treat that'll also provide you with the blood pressure–lowering electrolyte minerals calcium and potassium. I also like to spoon a generous heap of cocoa powder into the breakfast smoothies I've become addicted to. Take a look at my suggestions in the recipe section.

Depending on your time availability, lifestyle, and proclivities, think about making some desserts with cocoa. Imagine truly healthy, therapeutic taste treats. Who doesn't love brownies? Or cookies? And for something exotic, try mole sauce, also invented by the Aztecs centuries ago, in some Mexican dishes. I've added a few recipes at the end of the book.

When shopping for cocoa powder, though, be careful. Read those labels! You *don't* want ordinary cocoa mix, the kind that you simply mix with water. These types are loaded with sugar and some of the worst possible fats, the partially hydrogenated oils along with powdered milk. Instead, look for packages and canisters of pure, unadulterated cocoa powder. There are dozens of brands through the world. One of the most famous and popular is made by Droste in Holland. One tablespoon, containing 5 grams of cocoa and nothing but cocoa, has a mere 15 calories. Green & Black's Cocoa Powder is another delicious choice, a personal favorite of mine. Hershey's cocoa powder is the least expensive and is quite good. Go on an exploratory cocoa shopping trip to a few markets and pick up a few different brands. You'll find subtle differences in taste and piquancy.

As you've read, early research shows great promise for these secret weapons. In the coming months and years we can expect additional investigations, and knowledge will grow. I'd suggest that from time to time you visit my Web site, www.thehealthyheart.net, where I'll post the latest developments, new products, and cutting-edge information.

An even better way to stay up-to-date on all heart-health matters in detail, from blood pressure to cholesterol, is to subscribe to my quarterly publication, *The Diet-Heart Newsletter*. I've been particularly edified to learn that many physicians and other health-care professionals subscribe because they've found the newsletter to be the most convenient way for them to stay current on the newest research findings published in the various medical and nutrition journals, new products on the market, and insider reports from major scientific conferences around the world. To receive a free sample issue and subscription information, send a self-addressed, stamped, business-size envelope to: The Diet-Heart Newsletter, P.O. Box 2039, Venice, CA 90294.

15

The Blood Pressure Cure
Express Program

I've packed a lot of information about blood pressure and ways to control it in this book. But from time to time you may want to do a quick review or find the name and the Web site of a particular supplement or some other detail. That's why I've put together this summary of the entire Blood Pressure Cure program.

Blood Pressure: Definitions and Testing

Blood pressure is a measure of the force of blood rushing through and pushing against arteries. Measured in millimeters of mercury (mmHg), systolic blood pressure, the top number in, say, the reading 120/80, indicates arterial pressure as the heart beats, while the diastolic, the lower number, is the pressure between beats, while the heart rests.

Elevated levels of blood pressure constitute a major risk for cardiovascular disease, the number-one killer of both men and women. As with high cholesterol levels, there are no symptoms of high blood pressure, also termed hypertension.

Ideally, blood pressure should be no more than 120/80. When blood pressure increases to a range of 120–139/80–89, one is said to be in a state of prehypertension, a term that originated in 2003. Men and women with prehypertension are at some increased risk of cardiovascular disease, which could eventually lead to a heart attack or a stroke, and they are likely to see their blood pressure increase over the years unless they take steps to control it. Levels of 140/90 or more are considered to be hypertension. The higher blood pressure rises, the greater the risk.

Blood pressure testing in doctors' offices may be inaccurate owing to anxiety or other factors. For a diagnosis of hypertension, physicians take measurements on three separate visits with patients seated with feet on the floor, back supported in a chair, and relaxed. Today's home blood pressure monitoring devices have been shown to be as accurate as or even more accurate than in a doctor's office. A good brand to consider for your home is Omron; select a device with a cuff that goes around the upper arm rather than the wrist for greatest accuracy. I believe that home blood pressure monitors should be as common as scales.

Blood Pressure and Weight

Overweight and obesity predispose an individual to elevated blood pressure. It is important to try your very best to attain an ideal, healthy body weight. As a simple rule of thumb, men should have a waist circumference, a belt size, no greater than 40 inches and women no more than 32 inches.

Weight loss is not easy, but it can be achieved. As a first step, keep a daily journal of everything you eat and drink for a week. Read your journal and determine what foods and beverages are contributing excess calories and where you can cut back on those calories. Consider what I call preemptive snacking. Enjoy small, healthy snacks throughout the day so you never get so hungry that you overeat. Before heading out to a restaurant or a party, take the edge off your appetite so you'll eat smaller portions.

Blood Pressure–Friendly Foods

Several studies have come to the same conclusion that those who eat the most fruits and vegetables, whole-grain breads and cereals, small amounts of lean meats, fish, and poultry, and nonfat or low-fat dairy foods are least likely to develop hypertension. And by adopting that eating pattern you can significantly lower your blood pressure by as much as you might expect from a prescription blood pressure drug. The most well known of those studies is DASH (Dietary Approaches to Stop Hypertension).

Physical Activity

The Greek physician Hippocrates said it hundreds of years ago, though in more elegant terms: move it or lose it! An essential part of a heart-healthy lifestyle involves physical activity. That doesn't necessarily mean going to the gym, jogging, or other strenuous exercises you may not enjoy. The goal is a mere thirty minutes daily of simply moving around actively. That might mean taking a brisk walk, going dancing, gardening, or any other activity. Another way to look at it would be to shoot for walking ten thousand steps a day. You can do that with three ten-minute walks, taking the stairs rather than the elevator, or parking the car at the farthest end of the parking lot. Keep track of your daily steps with a good-quality pedometer such as the Yamax Digiwalker (find out more information at www.new-lifestyles.com or call 888-748-5377).

Coping with Stress

We all have stresses in our work, in our personal lives, and in ordinary, day-to-day activities such as driving in traffic. All stress and anger raise the heart rate and blood pressure, and those rises can become permanent. We can't rid ourselves of all stress, but we can learn to cope with it. One very efficient way is by increasing physical activity. Another is to take what I call mini-vacations, taking several minutes a few times a day, especially when stressed or angered, to simply close your eyes and concentrate on slow, rhythmic, deep breathing. Imagine your chest as a balloon you fill with air as fully as possible and then slowly deflate. RESPeRATE is a wonderful, clinically proven device to learn to control breathing, heart rate, and blood pressure. Learn more at www.resperate.com or call

877-988-9388. Also, consider taking one or two 100 mg capsules of L-theanine for a soothing, calming effect without side effects.

Salt and Sodium

We've heard a lot about how cutting back on salt and sodium is essential to blood pressure control. But take that advice with the proverbial grain of salt! Yes, very high salt and sodium intake can raise blood pressure. And extreme restriction can lower it. But this approach isn't practical, and many men and women are not sensitive to the effects of salt and sodium. By all means, we should practice moderation. But most of the sodium in the modern diet comes not from the salt shaker or the salt on the rim of a margarita glass but, rather, from processed and canned foods and from fast food.

Along with moderation, we can counterbalance sodium by increasing our consumption of the other mineral electrolytes—calcium, magnesium, and, especially, potassium. Shoot for a daily intake of about 4,500 mg of potassium by eating more fruits and vegetables and by adding a teaspoon or two of a salt substitute consisting of potassium chloride when cooking. Mushrooms and shellfish offer a lot of magnesium. Enjoy nonfat and low-fat dairy products or consider a daily supplement. Cal-Mag is a combination mineral supplement made by Endurance Products (www.endur.com or 800-483-2532).

Alcohol

Not long ago, doctors told patients fighting hypertension to avoid alcoholic beverages entirely. Today the word is moderation. In fact, one to two drinks daily can actually improve blood pressure levels. One for women, two for men. Overindulging can, in fact, aggravate blood pressure issues.

Don't Forget Cholesterol

Research shows that as we reduce elevated cholesterol levels, blood pressure comes down as well. That's a nice bonus, fighting two risk factors at once. Limit saturated and trans fats in your diet. Eat a lot of fruits, vegetables, and whole-grain breads and cereals. Enjoy plenty of the healthy fats, including olive oil, nuts of all kinds, avocados, and fish that provide heart-protecting omega-3 fatty acids. For those with a genetic predisposition to make too much cholesterol—80 percent of all the cholesterol in our bloodstream is produced in the liver—a better alternative to statin drugs are larger than nutritional doses of the vitamin niacin that both lowers the bad LDL cholesterol and raises the good HDL cholesterol. The plant sterols called phytosterols are also proven to lower cholesterol; find them in supplements or in fortified foods. Check out Endurance Products at www.endur.com or call 800-483-2532 for more information.

Five Secret Weapons against High Blood Pressure

Four supplements have been clinically proven to dramatically reduce blood pressure levels, producing results as good as would be expected from prescription antihypertensive drugs without the side effects. These four secret weapons, newly introduced to the market, include:

1. Sustained-release arginine, an amino acid that helps the body produce nitric oxide in the lining of the arteries. The nitric oxide relaxes the arteries, making them more elastic and flexible, thus allowing more efficient blood flow resulting in lower blood pressure. You can find EP Sustained-Release L-Arginine at www.endur.com or call 800-483-2532. Take three tablets in the morning and in the evening. Caution: Ordinary arginine in health food stores won't produce the desired effects because it does not remain in the bloodstream.
2. A specially formulated grape seed extract that concentrates the isolate clinically proven to bring blood pressure down. This is sold as MegaNatural-BP by Polyphenolics. Take one capsule daily at any time. You can find it at www.polyphenolics.com or call 866-308-7678. Again, standard formulations of grape seed extract are not expected to lower blood pressure.
3. Lyc-O-Mato, a tomato extract that Israeli researchers found in two studies to lower blood pressure in patients who were

currently taking antihypertensive drugs but were not at target levels and in patients who had never taken drugs for their elevated blood pressure levels. The dosage used in the studies was 15 mg daily, either at once or in divided amounts. While it contains the powerful antioxidant lycopene, that substance alone does not lower blood pressure. Visit www.lycomato.com or www.lycored.com for more information. You can also find Lyc-O-Mato at www.vitaminshoppe.com, 800-223-1216; www.swansonvitamins.com, 800-824-4491; and www.healthyorigins.com, 800-228-6650.

4. Pycnogenol, a particular formulation of French Maritime pine bark extract, which also has been proven in human clinical studies to effectively lower blood pressure. Only the French Maritime formulation has been tested, so other products containing pine bark extract may not work. The recommended dosage is 200 mg daily. To locate a number of Internet distributors of Pycnogenol, go to www.pycnogenol.com or call 877-369-9934.

To start, I'd recommend taking the sustained-release arginine and one of the other three supplements. Try them for six to eight weeks. If additional blood pressure reduction is needed, add one of the others. Or you could begin with all four and gradually cut back. In all cases, Arginine should be the backbone of the effort, in concert with one or more of the others.

The fifth of my secret weapons is a pure delight. Enjoy a relaxing mug of steaming, fragrant cocoa in the evening while winding down from the day, perhaps an hour or so before bedtime. Don't use the mixes that combine cocoa with sugar and various fats. Choose a brand of the darkest, richest cocoa you can find. The darker the cocoa, the more polyphenols it contains, and it's the polyphenols that have been clinically documented to reduce blood pressure. Mix a heaping tablespoon of cocoa with eight ounces of nonfat milk and the sweetener of your choice, heat it on the stove or in the microwave, and enjoy.

Best wishes for lower blood pressure and a healthy, happy heart!

16

Understanding Prescription Drugs: The Last Resort to Lowering Blood Pressure

Hypertension affects about one billion people worldwide. The higher the blood pressure, the greater your risk of having a heart attack, heart failure, a stroke, and kidney disease. Hypertension remains one of the Western world's major killers. These facts cannot be denied. Conversely, the more you can lower your blood pressure, the greater the reduction in your risk.

For many if not most men and women, following the programs and suggestions in this book will very effectively lower their blood pressure. The blood pressure–lowering effects can be similar to, if not even better than, those of potent prescription drugs when followed faithfully.

So why would I even bother to include a chapter dealing exclusively with those prescription drugs? There are two reasons. First, some individual cases of hypertension are so severe and life-threatening that one must use every option available. The person with a blood pressure of 225/115 is in immediate danger and must be given urgent attention. In such instances, resorting to prescription drugs may be unavoidable, and I would be wrong to argue against their use.

Second, not everyone is willing to make the lifestyle modifications I advocate and to take the nondrug supplements that I personally take and recommend. It truly troubles me to think about and admit it, but many people would rather take a pill prescribed by their physician than take personal responsibility. To make a comparison, dramatic cholesterol reductions are possible without the use of prescription drugs, but the cholesterol-lowering statin drugs remain best-sellers, making fortunes for the pharmaceutical companies.

If I were diagnosed with hypertension, I would ask my physician to allow me to have a trial period of lifestyle modification and supplements as detailed throughout this book. I know from personal experience with my fight against cholesterol that I would do my utmost to succeed in that trial. Unless my initial blood pressure was so high that even with my best efforts it remained at a dangerous level, I'm confident that the trial would be successful. But if I was starting with a degree of hypertension that, although lowered through such efforts, still posed a threat to my health, I'd very definitely work with my physician to find a drug or drugs that would lessen or eliminate the risk.

In the worst-case scenario, maximizing those lifestyle modifications and adding the blood pressure–lowering supplements would still have tremendous benefits even if I had to take one of those drugs. Simply enough, I would be able to minimize the dosage needed and thus limit the potential side effects and adverse reactions that universally accompany antihypertensive drugs.

Never forget that you are in partnership with your physician, that you have a say in the decision-making process, and that ultimately you will play a major role in your own health destiny. It is ironic that people will be more selective in choosing an auto mechanic than a physician! You owe it to yourself and your loved ones to find a doctor with whom you can establish an excellent personal relationship. Does your doctor fully answer your questions, consider your special needs and problems, and leave you with a sense of confidence? If not, find another doctor! If you have hypertension, controlling that condition will be a lifelong endeavor. And if you require antihypertensive drugs, a great deal of effort will go into the search for just the right drug and the proper dosage for you. You'll be spending quite a bit of time with your physician, so you'd better have a very good relationship with him or her!

The best patient is a well-informed patient. You need to know as much about your disease and potential therapies as possible. The world of antihypertensive drugs can at first appear bewildering. Having some knowledge about those drugs—and that doesn't mean you need to become a pharmacist—will help both you and your doctor successfully lower your blood pressure. So let's begin with a brief survey of the drug categories and how those medicines work.

Categories of Antihypertensive Drugs and Their Side Effects

Diuretics

The diuretic drugs lower blood pressure by helping the body to eliminate excessive fluids and sodium through urination. These are among the oldest and most established of all antihypertensive drugs. They are particularly effective for people who are sodium sensitive, individuals with a culturally high salt intake, and blacks. Diuretics are frequently prescribed as "first line" drugs and may be combined with one or two other blood pressure–lowering drugs. Certain diuretics, the thiazides, can act as vasodilators, opening blood vessels. Doctors may also suggest a high-potassium diet or may prescribe potassium supplements since the diuretics may reduce potassium levels too much.

Side effects include weakness; leg cramps; fatigue; (infrequently) gout; increased blood sugar, especially for people with diabetes; and reduced libido and/or impotence. The frequent need to urinate can be annoying.

Within the group, there are three subcategories:

Thiazide diuretics (Trade or brand names are given in parentheses.)
Chlorothiazide (Diuril)
Chlorthalidone (generic)
Hydrocholorothiazide (Microzide, HydroDiuril)

Polythiazide (Renese)

Indapamide (Lozol)

Metolazone (Mykrox) (This is not typically used for blood pressure control but rather as a very powerful diuretic for patients with refractory heart failure.)

Loop Diuretics (Trade or brand names are given in parentheses.)
Bumetanide (Bumex)
Furosemide (Lasix)
Torsemide (Demadex)

Potassium-Sparing Diuretics (Trade or brand names are given in parentheses. This category is not usually used for blood pressure control.)
Amiloride (Midamor)
Triamterene (Dyrenium)

Beta Blockers

The beta-blocking drugs, fully termed beta-adrenergic blockers, slow the heart rate and the amount of blood pumped, thus lowering blood pressure. They are routinely prescribed to patients following a heart attack (myocardial infarction or MI), since research has shown that taking these drugs for at least one year after an MI can help to prevent a second event. Beta blockers are also used to treat heartbeat disturbances called arrhythmias. They work by blocking the effects of heart-stimulating substances such as adrenaline, as well as by decreasing the production of adrenaline in the brain; therefore, they have a "central mediating" effect on blood pressure. These drugs are often used in combination with other antihypertensive agents.

Side effects include reduced exercise capacity, lethargy, fatigue, and impotence. Diabetics must have their insulin responses monitored regularly.

Following is a list of the more common beta blockers (trade names are given in parentheses).

Acebutolol (Sectral)
Atenolol (Tenormin)
Betaxolol (Kerlone)
Bisoprolol/hydrocholorothiazide (Ziac)
Bisoprolol (Zebeta)
Carteolol (Cartrol)
Metoprolol (Lopressor, Toprol XL)
Nadolol (Corgard)
Propranolol (Inderal)
Sotalol (Betapace)
Timolol (Blocadren)
Generic versions of the previously listed beta blockers are widely available.

ACE (Angiotensin-Converting Enzyme) Inhibitors

By blocking the action of the enzyme that activates angiotensin, which is involved with blood pressure control within the arteries, the ACE inhibitors prevent constriction of those blood vessels, instead causing dilation of the vessels and thus decreasing resistance to the flow of blood, which in turn lowers blood pressure.

Side effects may be a skin rash or other allergic reactions, a loss of taste, a chronic dry cough, and possibly kidney damage. That said, ACE inhibitors are generally well tolerated.

Following is a list of ACE inhibitors (trade or brand names are given in parentheses).

Benazepril (Lotensin)
Captopril (Capoten)
Enalapril (Vasotec)
Fosinopril (Monopril)
Lisinopril (Prinivil, Zestril)
Moexipril (Univasc)
Perindopril (Aceon)
Quinapril (Accupril)
Ramipril (Altace)
Trandolapril (Mavik)

Angiotensin-2 Receptor Antagonists (Blockers)

These rather new drugs, commonly referred to as ARBs, block the hormone that's responsible for constricting arteries and for making the kidneys retain more sodium and water. The action is similar to that of the ACE inhibitors, but instead of lowering levels of angiotensin-2 by blocking the needed enzyme, the drugs keep the chemical from having negative effects on the heart and the arteries. ARBs are frequently prescribed for patients who develop a cough from taking ACE inhibitors.

Side effects include headache, dizziness, and fatigue.

Following is a list of angiotensin-2 receptor antagonists (trade or brand names are in parentheses).

Candesartan (Atacand)
Eprosartan (Teveten)
Irbesartan (Avapro)
Losartan (Cozaar)
Telmisartan (Micardis)
Valsartan (Diovan)

Renin Inhibitor

Renin inhibitors comprise an entirely new category of drugs that target the very beginning of the renin/angiotensin system in the kidneys. This system is one of the two major factors influencing blood pressure. Renin is an enzyme that converts the substance angiotensinogen to angiotensin, which influences blood pressure. Rather than interfering with either angiotensinogen or angiotensin as do the previous two categories of drugs, the renin inhibitors, as the name suggests, deter overproduction of renin. As a result there is less angiotensinogen and less angiotensin and subsequently less effect on elevating blood pressure. Doctors are pretty excited about this drug made by the Novartis pharmaceutical company under the trade name Rasilex (aliskiren). In simplest terms, Rasilex gets right to the heart of the problem, at the start of the process in the kidneys that leads to elevations in blood pressure. And medical authorities believe that this drug can also help to protect the kidney itself.

Rasilex is a very potent and effective antihypertensive drug, based on clinical trials that have been conducted in the United States and elsewhere. It can be used alone or in combination with other drugs, or with the secret weapon supplements, if additional blood pressure reduction is necessary. Currently, Rasilex is the only drug in the renin inhibitor class; additional agents probably will not be available until approximately 2012.

I am particularly interested in Rasilex and am delighted to see its availability for those men and women with very high blood pressure who may not respond adequately to the secret weapons alone or in conjunction with the entire program in this book. Why am I so enthusiastic about a drug? Rasilex does not affect physiological and biochemical responses that are responsible for the dry cough, edema, and buildup of watery fluid, often associated with the ACE inhibitors.

Talk with your doctor about whether this new drug might be helpful in your particular case and how you might use it in conjunction with the secret weapon supplements as well as the entire Blood Pressure Cure program.

Calcium Channel Blockers

This category of antihypertensive agents, also called calcium antagonists, interrupts the passage of calcium into heart and arterial muscle cells. This restricts arterial constriction, allowing for greater ease of blood flow and thus lowering blood pressure. Physicians also prescribe the calcium channel blockers to treat heartbeat irregularities and the chest pain known as angina pectoris (commonly called angina).

Side effects include palpitations of the heart, swollen ankles, a rash, constipation, headaches, and dizziness. Different drugs within the category may be more prone to causing particular side effects than others are. Ask your doctor about this if he or she prescribes one of the following drugs.

Following is a list of calcium channel blockers (trade or brand names are in parentheses).

Amlodipine (Norvasc, Lotrel)
Bepridil (Vascor)
Diltiazem (Cardizem, Tiazac)

Felodipine (Plendil)
Nifedipine (Adalat, Procardia)
Nimodipine (Nimotop)
Nisoldipine (Sular)
Verapamil (Calan, Isoptin, Verelan)

Alpha Blockers

This group of drugs selectively blocks particular blood chemicals that cause arteries to constrict. Blocking them allows for greater blood flow and lowered blood pressure by relaxing the arteries.

Side effects include lightheadedness or dizziness, sleepiness, increased heart rate, or a blood pressure drop that produces dizziness when you get up from a chair or a bed.

Following is a list of alpha blockers (trade or brand names are in parentheses).

Doxazosin (Cardura)
Prazosin (Minipress)
Terazosin (Hytrin)

Combined Alpha and Beta Blockers

These drugs provide the benefits of both alpha and beta inhibition and are used by someone who has suffered damage to the heart muscle from a heart attack.

Carvedilol (Coreg)
Labetalol (Normodyne, Trandate)

The most typical side effect is dizziness when you stand up from a sitting or lying position, caused by a drop in blood pressure. This is termed *postural hypotension* or *orthostatic hypotension*. Adjusting the dosage may help.

Central Alpha-2 Agonists

Also called centrally acting alpha agents, this category of drugs is very different from others in that these drugs act in the brain, where they switch off brain activity that constricts arteries.

The most common side effects within this category are sleepiness and sexual dysfunction. Side effects vary by subcategory, and I've noted them below the following list of centrally acting alpha agents (trade or brand names are in parentheses).

Clonidine (Catapres) (also available as a patch)
Guanabenz (Wytensin)
Guanfacine (Tenex)

The previously listed three drugs have the potential of causing severe mouth dryness, drowsiness, or constipation. But if you develop any of these side effects, don't stop taking the drug suddenly, as your blood pressure could rapidly soar to dangerous levels. Speak with your doctor.

Alpha methyldopa (Aldomet)

This drug may lower your blood pressure so much that when you stand or walk, you might feel weak or may even faint. It can also cause sleepiness, sluggishness, dry mouth, fever, and anemia. Men may experience impotence. Work with your doctor to adjust the dosage to reduce those side effects as much as possible.

Dilating Drugs

As the name implies, these drugs open arteries by relaxing muscles in the walls of the vessels, allowing greater blood flow and reducing blood pressure.

Hydralazine (Apresoline)

Side effects include headaches, swelling around the eyes, heart palpitations, and joint pain or achiness. These effects may lessen after you take the drug for a few weeks.

Minoxidil (Loniten)

Doctors typically reserve this potent drug for patients with extremely high blood pressure that has not responded to lesser therapies. It may cause excessive hair growth and/or significant weight gain owing to water retention. The hair growth side effect was noted by the company that developed the drug, and it subsequently sold a greatly reduced dosage as an over-the-counter treatment for male balding.

Combination Therapies

Most typically, it will take two, three, or even four different drugs, working in various ways as described previously, to achieve adequate blood pressure control. Some available medications combine two drug types, such as an ACE inhibitor and a thiazide diuretic, in one tablet or capsule. Certain doctors like to offer their patients the convenience, while others prefer to customize the combination. Following are some of the available combination drugs.

> Benazepril and hydrochlorothiazide (Lotensin)
> Enalapril and hydrochlorothiazide (Vaseretic)
> Lisinopril and hydrochlorothiazide (Prinzide and Zestoretic)
> Moexipril and hydrochlorothiazide (Uniretic)
> Quinapril and hydrochlorothiazide (Accuretic)

British medical authorities got a lot of media attention when they proposed a "polypill" that would combine a cholesterol-lowering drug and two blood pressure medications. Their rationale was that many patients have both elevated cholesterol and high blood pressure, so giving a single pill could potentially prevent many heart attacks, strokes, and deaths.

While that particular combination isn't currently on the market, one product (Caduet) combines Lipitor (atorvastatin) for cholesterol lowering and Norvasc (amlodipine) for blood pressure reduction. Caduet is available in a wide variety of dosages of both agents, allowing physicians to choose the one that would best suit a particular patient. That's much better than a fixed combination, since typically one size does *not* fit all.

Which Drug Is Best?

This question might seem fairly straightforward, but it is highly controversial. Studies have been published and widely publicized in the medical community that come to very different conclusions. Some doctors say always to start with a diuretic and add other drugs as needed. Other doctors prefer to initiate therapy with an ACE inhibitor. Often, cost is offered as a rationale. According to one major medical group, "Fewer than 50 percent of patients treated for hypertension will achieve an optimal blood pressure response with a single agent (monotherapy). In the majority of cases a combination of antihypertensive drugs from two or more antihypertensive drug classes will therefore be required."

One of the most cited studies, the Antihypertensive and Lipid-Lowering Treatment to Prevent Heart Attack Trial (ALLHAT), concluded that the thiazide-type diuretics are "unsurpassed in lowering blood pressure, reducing clinical events, and tolerability, and less costly." Results of that study, familiar to all physicians who treat hypertension, were published in 2002. The same conclusion was reached in 2006 by researchers at the University of Texas who noted the superiority of diuretics over calcium channel blockers and ACE inhibitors in treating hypertension and preventing heart failure. It's worth noting that about two of every three patients in ALLHAT needed two or more drugs to achieve blood pressure control of less than 140/90. Patients in that study were older than fifty-five years of age and one-third were African Americans; both groups are most likely to respond to thiazide medications. Literally dozens of studies have been published, often with varying conclusions. The Australian National Blood Pressure 2 study demonstrated the benefits of ACE inhibitors. That was also the case in the European Heart Outcomes Prevention Evaluation (HOPE) study, which specifically worked with the ACE inhibitor ramipril (Altace).

Doctors look to the medical literature for guidance but often find conflicting information and data. For example, a study funded by the U.S. National Heart, Lung, and Blood Institute found that diuretic drugs work as well or better than Norvasc in protecting against heart attacks and strokes. The cost of a diuretic drug, widely available in generic forms, is a fraction of that of Norvasc.

Conversely, the much-touted ASCOT (Anglo-Scandinavian Cardiac Outcomes Trial) study found that treating with beta blockers, diuretics, or both increased the risk of developing diabetes by about 40 percent and had some other side effects as well.

Certain population groups are also served better by particular drugs. Studies have found and physicians have observed over the years that people who are sodium sensitive and/or who are members of an ethnic group such as African Americans whose diet is heavy on salt will frequently do best with diuretic drugs, calcium channel blockers, or both.

The beta-blocker drug atenolol has long been viewed as sort of a gold standard in comparison with other antihypertensive agents and has been prescribed frequently by physicians as the drug to start newly diagnosed hypertensive patients on. But studies of late have cast a shadow on atenolol, showing no particular benefit in terms of blood pressure–lowering advantage and a less-than-desired ability to prevent heart attacks and strokes.

Patients most often have more than one medical problem at a time. For people suffering from mitral valve disease along with hypertension, ACE inhibitors seem to be a good choice, but they're not for anyone who has valvular disease and normal blood pressure.

Diabetic individuals pose an entirely different challenge to physicians. They are at a much higher risk of developing cardiovascular disease, and blood pressure targets for diabetics are significantly lower than for people without that disease.

The Australian Heart Foundation provides the following guidelines for physicians in determining *potentially unfavorable effects* on coexisting conditions:

Coexisting Condition	Drug Not Recommended
Asthma	Beta blockers
Low heart rate (bradycardia)	Beta blockers, calcium channel blockers
Diabetes	Beta blockers, diuretics
Gout	Thiazide diuretics
Heart failure	Calcium channel blockers, alpha blockers
Kidney disease, pregnancy	ACE inhibitors, ARBs
Peripheral vascular disease (atherosclerosis in the leg arteries)	Beta blockers

The United States and New Zealand are the only two countries that permit drug advertising by pharmaceutical companies. That's good for the rest of the world, but bad for our two countries. Those TV ads often provide misleading information in the rosiest possible tones, promising great results without disclosing the full picture, and they urge viewers to "talk with your doctor" about this drug or that. Doctors often feel pressured by patients coming into the office with demands for particular drugs, putting the credibility of a thirty-second TV spot or a magazine ad ahead of a physician's decades of medical training and years of experience with patients.

Ultimately, the decision must be made by your personal physician, taking into consideration your unique medical history and patient profile. Assuming that you have confidence in your physician—something I believe is essential—trust his or her judgment, but be sure to communicate effectively. Let your doctor know about any and all side effects that crop up. Remember always, however, that you must not abruptly stop taking any antihypertensive drug, since that could result in a severe change in blood pressure that could be very dangerous, if not actually life threatening.

No single drug will completely cure hypertension, and no doctor will disagree with that. Proper treatment, if indeed drug therapy is needed, must also include aggressive lifestyle modification for best results. That includes weight control, moderation in alcohol consumption, giving up smoking, increased physical activity, and stress management. Without such efforts, your chances of attaining optimal blood pressure are greatly reduced. As my last thought in this paragraph, although prescription drugs for blood pressure control can have side effects, these are not experienced by all patients. Again, by working closely with your physician you can have the best of both worlds: blood pressure control with the fewest possible adverse effects.

17

Recipes for Healthy
Blood Pressure

I am not now, nor have I ever been, a member of the Food Police! These are the health zealots whose food philosophy can be summarized simply as follows: if it tastes good, spit it out. I happen to love food, and I believe that truly delicious food can also be good for your health.

In 1987, I introduced the notion that certain foods could actually lower cholesterol, thereby protecting the heart. The soluble fiber in oats and beans reduces LDL cholesterol without lowering the protective HDL, and fish oils prevent excessive blood clot production. Similarly, certain foods and recipes that contain soluble fiber can actively affect blood pressure. I've included some representative recipes in this chapter to inspire you to eat more fruits and vegetables, especially those rich in potassium, such as sweet potatoes, bananas, and mangos, and more seafood, which not only affects blood clot formation but also lowers blood pressure.

If you traveled to Italy, Spain, the south of France, Greece, and throughout Asia, you'd enjoy the wonderful native cuisines. Those foods happen to be some of the best in the world for heart health in general and for blood pressure control in particular. As an appetizer in Italy you might munch on bruschetta, crusty bread topped with olive oil, garlic, and chopped tomatoes and basil. In

Spain you might have a salad of roasted bell peppers sprinkled with capers and a bit of crumbled cheese. How could you visit Marseilles in France without sitting down to a bowl of steaming bouillabaise?

Then, if you're like most people, you'd come home and return to your old eating habits. Who'd think of making bruschetta? Or bell pepper salad? Or bouillabaise? Or any number of wonderful dishes that your heart would thank you for? Too much work, you might think. Not enough time to prepare. I hope to change your mind in this chapter, to share with you some of my favorite foods, and to show you how easy it is to enjoy a wide variety of heart-healthy foods on a regular basis.

Obviously, this is not a cookbook. I'd just like to give you some ideas that could perk up your taste buds while bringing down your blood pressure. Since the research data are so convincing that a diet rich in fruits and vegetables contributes to healthy blood pressure levels, I'm going to stress those foods. I think you will surprise yourself by actually enjoying fruits and vegetables more than you thought possible. All I ask is that you give some of these ideas a chance.

I really believe that Americans eat so few fruits and vegetables because they don't know what to do with them beyond simply peeling a banana or boiling a bunch of carrots. Pretty boring for the most part. Sure, a nice ripe banana can be a quick, tasty snack, but very little effort converts that humble banana into a spectacular flaming dessert. And those carrots come alive with flavor after adding a touch of this and a sprig of that.

I also know that few of us have the time or the inclination to follow complicated directions in recipes. While I have an entire library of cookbooks, most of the time I cook with no recipe at all. I just throw a bit of this and that together, spending as little time cooking as possible. Sure, what I'm about to put into this book are "recipes," but I'm hoping you'll use them more as suggestions rather than following them to the letter.

Try to taste the foods as you read about them. It's difficult to think about slicing into a juicy lemon without the thought making your mouth water. With a little practice you can accurately predict how a dish will taste when you prepare it. If you see something in one of my suggestions that you dislike, simply avoid that ingredient. Conversely, if you see an ingredient you really like, you might want to double the amount I recommend. I do that most of the time when a recipe calls for garlic. No vampires in my house!

I'll start with a story I like to tell about a cooking class my wife and I took at a French restaurant years ago when we lived in Chicago. The little bistro was owned and operated by a husband and wife team, Renee and Josie, who both cooked and loved food. Josie stressed the notion of simply looking around at what you have in your kitchen and coming up with something delicious to eat.

As an example, one evening she took an orange and said it would be a good start for a dessert. She sliced off the rind, cut the orange into quarter rounds, placed those slices on a plate, sprinkled them with a tiny amount of brown sugar, and then drizzled some dark rum over them to complete the delicious treat. Josie passed the plate around for us to taste, and the whole class loved it. There you have it: a recipe in just one sentence. You won't even have to pull this book out when you want to make this quick and easy dessert. You could even dress it up for company with a few sprigs of mint. Do you have young children in your family? Drizzle their orange slices with alcohol-free rum extract.

Some of the recipes in the coming pages will be just that simple, while others will have step-by-step instructions and lists of ingredients. But even recipes in the latter category will be so easy that after the first preparation, you'll probably have them memorized such that you'll be able to throw them together the next time.

I have not provided nutrition information for the recipes in this chapter. Why? None of the recipes contain the fats you should avoid, and all of them provide the nutrients that are essential for good heart health while being very low in calories. Don't worry about numbers. Just eat good foods.

Salads

MEDITERRANEAN/GREEK SALAD

With few variations, this is the staple salad whether you're in Greece or elsewhere in the Mediterranean.

Start with a cucumber and a tomato, more than one of each if you're preparing the salad for more than two people or if you'd like leftovers. I prefer to peel the cuke, although some folks don't. Or you could get fancy and run a fork's tines down the length of it to score the skin. One way or the other, slice the cucumber lengthwise into quarters, then cut it into bite-size chunks. Do the same with the tomato. Mix them with oil and vinegar or a bottled dressing of your choice. You can add a few sprigs of mint if you like; that's the way they do it in some countries. Chill the salad in the refrigerator. Serve it with crumbled low-fat feta cheese.

TRI-COLOR ROASTED BELL PEPPER SALAD

At first reading, you might think this salad is complicated and diffi-cult, but if you try it you'll not only love it but you'll also see how simple it is to prepare.

Start with three bell peppers: red, yellow, and orange. Cut off the tops, slice each pepper in half, and remove the seeds and mem-branes inside. Flatten the pepper halves, arrange them on a cookie pan or a broiler pan, and place the pan under the broiler in the oven. Broil them until the skins are completely blackened, remove them from the oven, and place them in a plastic bag for about an hour. By the time the roasted peppers are cool, you'll be able to eas-ily remove the blackened skins. Rinse them under running water.

Arrange pieces of the three different-colored peppers on salad greens on individual plates, drizzle everything with a little good olive oil, and scatter a few capers and a bit of crumbled feta or blue cheese over the top. Enjoy the salad with a crusty chunk of bread. This is festive enough for company, a truly attractive dish, and something you can prepare an hour or so before your guests arrive.

GREENS, CHEESE, AND PEPPERED HONEY SALAD

The name says it all.

On one side of each individual plate, pile some seasonal wild greens. The other side of the plate gets a thin slice of the cheese of your choice. It could be a low-fat mozzarella, feta, or fontina. I use whatever happens to be in the refrigerator at the time. Dribble honey over the cheese and the greens and coarsely grind pepper over them. Or if someone in the family dislikes pepper, as my wife, Dawn, does, skip that for his or her plate, although I personally think the combined tastes of honey and pepper are a wonderful and delightful surprise. I first enjoyed this salad in a restaurant, paid ten dollars for it, and thought, "Hey, I can do this!"

HONEYDEW MELON AND AVOCADO WITH HONEY/LIME DRESSING

To fully enjoy this salad, wait until the time of year when honeydew melons and avocados are in season and are most juicy, sweet, and flavorful.

Arrange alternate slices of melon and avocado over a few leaves of romaine lettuce. Blend equal amounts of honey and lime juice (fresh juice tastes best, of course) in a measuring cup. The juice cuts the honey and makes a wonderful dressing for the salad. It's best if all the ingredients are chilled in advance.

THREE-BEAN SALAD

I think every family in America has a favorite recipe for this classic salad, which is so frequently brought to summer picnics, but I think this one that I learned from a neighbor is best.

⅓ cup granulated sugar
½ cup canola oil
¾ cup red wine vinegar
1 teaspoon salt
16-ounce can cut green beans, drained

16-ounce can garbanzo beans, drained
16-ounce can kidney beans, drained
½ cup red onions, chopped

Combine the sugar, oil, vinegar, and salt in a large bowl. Add the beans and onions and toss to coat them thoroughly. Refrigerate them in a large, covered container at least overnight. Stir the salad once or twice to develop the full flavor.

RED POTATO SALAD

Potatoes are great sources of potassium, and keeping the skins on preserves both the fiber and the nutrients in this recipe. Use whole eggs if you're taking phytosterols to block dietary cholesterol. Otherwise, you can use egg whites. During the summer, I love this salad with hamburgers made on the grill.

5 pounds red potatoes (pick the smallest ones)	12 hard-cooked egg whites, or 6 whole eggs
salt (optional)	12 large green olives with pimentos
2 medium green bell peppers (or 1 green and 1 red)	low-fat mayonnaise
5 stalks celery	paprika

Boil the potatoes in their skins in water (salted, in you prefer) for about 15 minutes, or until they're barely tender. While the potatoes cook, dice the peppers, celery, and eggs and slice the pimentos. Allow the potatoes to cool, then cut them into chunks. Mix all the ingredients with mayonnaise to taste. Sprinkle the potato salad with paprika.

SWEET POTATO SALAD

Try this one for something different. It works really well with turkey roasted over the coals. Serve it with cranberry sauce on the side. American Thanksgiving in the summer!

2 large sweet potatoes (yams)	2 tablespoons lemon juice
1 cup celery (4 to 5 stalks), diced	2 tablespoons sugar
1 cup apples, diced	salt (optional)
⅓ cup walnuts, chopped	low-fat mayonnaise

Cut the sweet potatoes into chunks with the skins left on to pre-serve the fiber and nutrients. Bring them to a boil in water (salted, if you prefer) and cook them until tender but not soft. While cook-ing the potatoes, prepare the other ingredients. When the potatoes are cool, mix all the ingredients with mayonnaise to taste.

CARROT SALAD

1 pound carrots, shredded
½ cup raisins
½ cup celery, diced
1 teaspoon lemon juice
1 teaspoon granulated sugar
low-fat mayonnaise

Nothing difficult about this one. Simply mix all the ingredients together with mayonnaise to taste. Shred the carrots by hand or with a food processor; or make it easy on yourself and buy shred-ded carrots at the supermarket.

COLONEL KOWALSKI'S COLESLAW

This is my version of KFC's slaw. The trick is to chop the cabbage and carrots into tiny bits. I like the clean, crisp taste. It goes well with sandwiches of all sorts, adding the veggies we don't normally get at lunch. Chop, mix, chill, and serve.

8 cups cabbage (use either stan-dard green cabbage or half and half red), chopped
1 cup carrots, chopped
½ cup granulated sugar
salt (optional)
¼ teaspoon ground white pepper
½ cup low-fat mayonnaise
½ cup low-fat buttermilk
1½ tablespoons white vinegar
2½ tablespoons lemon juice

HEALTHY HOLLYWOOD COBB SALAD

I was lucky enough to move to Los Angeles just before the famous Brown Derby restaurant closed. The Cobb salad invented there has gone on for decades because it's so delicious. I like this vegetarian version because it's one of the easiest ways to get plenty of veggies of all sorts. Make a big bag full and keep it in the refrigerator.

2 cups mixed greens, chopped
½ cup each: mushrooms, broccoli,
   carrots, all chopped

¼ cup each: sweet onions, beets,
   bell peppers, all chopped

Combine all the ingredients and mix them well in a large plastic bag. Keep them chilled until you're ready to serve the salad with the dressing of your choice. This recipe is enough for two people. Multiply the ingredients for larger groups or to keep it on hand. Top the salad off with sliced grilled chicken or salmon and you have a complete, wonderful meal. Or put the chopped veggies in a sliced roll for a salad sandwich.

Soups to Warm Your Soul and Nourish Your Heart

MINESTRONE SOUP

There are as many recipes for minestrone soup as there are Italian restaurants. Everyone has a favorite, and this is one of mine. Eat it in place of a salad at the start of a meal, or, for a satisfying meal, have a large bowl with a chunk of crusty Italian bread and a glass of red wine. Please don't let the long list of ingredients put you off. You can't fail.

1 medium onion, minced
1 scallion, minced
2 teaspoons olive oil
2 medium carrots, peeled and
   diced
2 quarts low-sodium chicken broth
2 red potatoes, diced with skins
   left on
1 can white or kidney beans,
   drained and rinsed
2 small zucchini, diced
2 celery stalks, diced
1 tablespoon tomato paste
½ small head of cabbage, finely
   chopped

½ tablespoon Italian seasoning
2 bay leaves
4 ounces elbow macaroni
1 can low-sodium whole
   Italian tomatoes, cut into
   chunks
1 package frozen spinach
½ cup frozen peas
3 tablespoons parsley (Italian
   broad leaf, if available),
   chopped
salt (optional)
½ teaspoon fresh ground black
   pepper

Sauté the onion and scallion in the olive oil for about 3 minutes in a large pot. Add the carrots and sauté for another 3 minutes. Add the broth and all the ingredients except the peas, parsley, tomatoes, spinach, and macaroni. Bring everything to a boil, lower the heat, and simmer the soup for 1 hour. Add the macaroni, tomatoes, spinach, peas, and parsley and simmer the soup for 10 minutes more. Add salt and pepper to taste. You'll find that this is even more delicious the next day after all the flavors merge.

JENNY'S BUTTERNUT SQUASH SOUP

My daughter, Jenny, makes, I think, the best butternut squash soup you'll ever eat. This is definitely worth your while to prepare. Make enough for leftovers, or make a double batch and freeze half for another time.

2 pounds butternut squash	¾ teaspoon curry powder
2 cups onion, chopped	¼ teaspoon each: ground nutmeg,
2 tablespoons olive oil	white pepper, ground ginger
4 cups low-sodium chicken broth	2 bay leaves
salt (optional)	½ cup low-fat sour cream

Preheat the oven to 350 degrees F. Cut the squash in half and scoop out the seeds. Place the halves in a casserole dish, cut side down, in about 1 inch of water. Bake the squash for 40 to 45 minutes. Allow it to cool, then remove the skin and cut the squash into chunks. (Prepare the other ingredients while the squash is baking.)

Sauté the onion in olive oil until it's transparent, 3 to 4 minutes. Stir in the chunks of squash, chicken broth, and seasonings. Bring this to a boil in a suitably sized pot, reduce the heat, and simmer it for 15 minutes.

Remove the bay leaves and blend the soup in a food processor or a blender in batches. Jenny finds that a hand mixer works well also. Return the soup to the pot, heat it through, and add the sour cream.

CREAM OF VEGETABLE SOUP

This is a basic recipe for making any kind of cream of vegetable soup, simply alternating the vegetable(s) you'd like to use that day. This is a good example of how once you make it, you'll never have to look at the recipe again. You'll just throw the ingredients together and it'll be done. Nothing to it at all.

4 cups cauliflower or broccoli florets, asparagus, carrots, or blend of root vegetables	2 bay leaves
	½ teaspoon ground white pepper
	½ teaspoon tarragon
4 cups low-sodium chicken, vegetable, or beef broth (try them all for variety)	½ teaspoon thyme
	1 cup low-fat sour cream

This is the essence of simplicity. Just put all the ingredients (except the sour cream) in a large pot, bring it to a boil, reduce it to a strong simmer, and cook the vegetables until they're very tender, almost mushy. Remove the bay leaves. Allow the soup to cool for easier handling. Blend it in a food processor or a blender in batches. Return the soup to the pot and heat it through. Blend in the sour cream.

GREENS AND BROTH

Every nutritionist says we should eat more leafy green vegetables such as escarole, spinach, and so on. But few people actually like greens very much. Instead of serving those greens on the plate as vegetables, I like to make them into a simple soup. This isn't my invention; it's the way Italians have cooked for decades.

Buy a bunch of greens at the supermarket and clean them under running water to get rid of any dirt and grit. Put them into a pot and pour in enough low-sodium broth (vegetable or chicken) to barely cover the greens. Flavor them with Italian seasoning and fresh ground pepper. Experiment with other herbs. Cook until the greens are tender—that doesn't take too long, so don't go read a book! Serve the greens in bowls as a side dish for the meal.

If you have a little more time and want to get fancy, start by sautéing two or three peeled garlic cloves in a tablespoon of olive oil until they're tender and translucent (never until they're brown, since garlic turns bitter). Then add the greens and chicken or vegetable broth. When the broth comes to a boil, add a half can of drained and rinsed Italian white beans (cannelloni), heat everything thoroughly, and serve. As the Italians say, "Mangiamo!"

Vegetable Side Dishes

BRUSCHETTA

You can enjoy this as a starter before the meal or along with it. What we have here is a combination, quite literally, of bread and veggies. Make it once and it'll be as much a part of your cuisine as it is in Italy. You'll laugh when you see it outrageously priced in restaurants.

Start with four large slices of good bread and toast them either in a toaster or under the broiler in the oven. While they're toasting, peel four garlic cloves. Then run the cloves over the toasted bread. The garlic will shred right into the bread as if it were sandpaper. Drizzle your best extra-virgin olive oil over the bread. Then top the bread with chopped, seeded Italian tomatoes and minced fresh basil leaves. That's it. Enjoy!

ACORN SQUASH

1 medium to large acorn squash for two people	1 tablespoon tub margarine
	2 tablespoons brown sugar

Cut the squash in half lengthwise and remove the seeds and membranes. Pierce the flesh of the squash repeatedly with a fork, taking care not to cut through the skin. Use your fingers to smear the inside of the squash halves with margarine, then sprinkle on the brown sugar. Microwave them for 12 to 15 minutes. Allow them to cool for ease of handling, then use a tablespoon to remove the squash meat from the skin, mixing in the margarine and sugar as you do so. Return the squash to the skins and reheat them in the microwave when you're ready to serve them.

ROASTED ROOT (AND OTHER) VEGETABLES

Don't you get sick and tired of just steaming or boiling vegetables? Of course, you do. That's one of the main reasons why we don't eat enough vegetables. Here's an easy-to-make change of pace that you and your family will love. And so will your heart.

Start with the root vegetables that fill supermarkets in the fall and throughout the winter. Peel four medium carrots, one parsnip, one turnip, and one rutabaga and cut them into medium-size pieces. Place them all in a plastic bag, pour in two tablespoons of olive oil, and sprinkle in just a pinch of salt, some fresh ground pepper, and ½ tablespoon of tarragon. Mix everything well so that the veggies are coated with the oil and seasonings. Arrange them in a single layer on an oven-safe casserole dish. Roast them at 350 degrees F for about 15 minutes or until they're tender. (My wife likes her vegetables crunchier and I prefer mine cooked through.)

You can use essentially the same technique for other vegetables as well. Asparagus stalks are particularly delicious roasted in that fashion, as is broccoli. You can add some minced garlic cloves to the asparagus. Also try beets. To roast potatoes, cut them in chunks with the skins still on and boil them for a few minutes to soften them a bit before putting them in the oven.

CARROTS AND DILL OR PARSLEY

Instead of buying beta-carotene supplements, eat more carrots and other yellow and orange vegetables such as squash. I'll bet you didn't know that beta-carotene is only one of more than five hundred carotenoids found in carrots. Why settle for just one?

Start with a bunch of carrots. My favorites are the ones with the greens still attached. Don't worry about quantity, since leftovers are never a problem. Make plenty. Just peel the carrots (or simply scrub them with a clean brush under running water) and cut them into rounds. Instead of using salt in enough water to cover them in a small pot, try a heaping tablespoon of granulated or brown sugar. They taste so much better that way, and you get rid of some sodium in your diet. I also like to add ¼ teaspoon of a salt substitute to boost my potassium intake. Bring them to a boil and simmer them until they're as tender as you like.

While the carrots are cooking, mince about a quarter cup of either fresh dill or parsley.

As a side note, I love the quote from the famed chef and cookbook author Julia Child, who said, "If you don't want to cook vegetables till they're tender, eat crudités!" Crudités, of course, are a platter of raw veggies served before dinner or at cocktail parties.

Anyway, once the carrots are tender, drain the water and put in a tablespoon of margarine and the minced dill or parsley. You'll fall in love with carrots again.

ROASTED TOMATOES

Just slice a tomato or two in half, scatter a few shreds of fresh basil on each half, and top them with parmesan cheese. Put the tomato halves in the oven or a roaster oven for about 15 minutes or until the cheese is melted and the tomato is cooked through. This is rich in nutrients, simple to prepare, and absolutely delicious as a side dish with almost any meal.

LEMON BROCCOLI

Plan on using about a pound of broccoli florets for four people. Place them in a shallow pan of water, bring it to a boil, reduce the heat to a simmer while the pan is covered, and cook the florets until they're bright green and done to your desired degree of tenderness. While the broccoli cooks, mix the juice of one-half lemon (a little more than 1 tablespoon), 1 tablespoon of olive oil, and ¼ teaspoon of ground white pepper in a little dish. Drain the broccoli and drizzle the lemon/oil mixture over it.

SAUTÉED GARLIC SPINACH

Here's a delicious way to get more leafy greens into our diets.

Plan on one bunch of spinach for a true spinach lover who's really hungry or for two more typical people. The most difficult part of spinach preparation is cleaning the leaves. I first rinse the bunch under running water to get rid of the dirt and grit, then put the leaves in a sink filled with cool water and swirl them around. Because I'm a picky eater, I take the time to pinch off the stems so that I get only the tender leaves. Or, you could take the easy way out and simply buy a package of prewashed, prepicked spinach— although I'd still recommend that you do at least a quick rinse.

Use either a salad spinner or kitchen towels to dry the leaves. (They don't have to be bone dry.)

Peel and mince several garlic cloves. My wife and I love garlic, so I plan on four cloves per bunch. Put the minced garlic in a fairly large pan that has a top and very gently sauté it in 2 tablespoons of good olive oil, just until the garlic is transparent. Don't let it get browned, since that makes garlic bitter. Next, dump the spinach in the pan and cover it. Put the pan on very low heat for just a few minutes, tossing the spinach now and then to make sure it's nicely coated with the garlicky olive oil. Serve and enjoy.

SIMPLE SPINACH

People often dislike spinach because it tastes bland. There's no reason for that.

Start your garlic preparation as in the previous sautéed spinach recipe, but don't bother to dry the leaves. Just dump the spinach into a large covered pot and cook it over a low heat. The moisture on the washed leaves will be enough to steam the spinach.

Serve it with a splash of balsamic or rice vinegar for a flavor treat. Or try something that my Dad introduced me to: sprinkle the spinach with a little sugar. It sounds weird, but it's really good.

GREEN BEANS WITH TOMATO SAUCE

This recipe is so good that my mouth is actually watering as I write it down even though I just finished breakfast this morning. It's very flavorful yet simple to prepare.

1 pound fresh green beans, cut into 2-inch lengths	1 tablespoon olive oil
3 garlic cloves	1 cup low-sodium tomato sauce
	1 tablespoon parmesan cheese

Gently boil the beans in a pot of water for about 8 minutes or until tender. (This would be another good time to add a quarter teaspoon of salt substitute to get more potassium.) While the beans are cooking, peel and mince the garlic cloves and sauté them in a pan with the olive oil. As soon as the garlic is transparent, not browned, add the tomato sauce and heat everything through. Drain the beans, add the garlic tomato sauce, put the beans into a serving dish, and sprinkle on the parmesan cheese.

SAUTÉED ONIONS AND PEPPERS

Did you know that bell peppers, especially the yellow and the red ones, have two to three times the vitamin C of oranges? They're also a pretty good source of potassium.

2 cloves of garlic	1 teaspoon Italian seasoning
2 tablespoons olive oil	¼ teaspoon red cayenne pepper
1 green and one yellow, orange, or red bell pepper, sliced into strips	(optional if you don't like the "bite" of pepper)
1 medium sweet onion, cut into half circles	

Sauté the garlic in olive oil in a skillet until it's barely transparent. Scoop out the garlic and reserve it. Sauté the peppers and onions until they're tender. Add the garlic, Italian seasoning, and pepper and heat everything through. The dish is colorful and delicious!

GRILLED EGGPLANT

Ordinarily, I don't like eggplant very much, and the odds are that you don't, either. But I cooked this for Dawn because she loves the stuff. Son of a gun, it was really good. Try this as an accompaniment to another grilled food, especially fish. That way, you can prepare both of them at the same time.

Start with a large, firm eggplant to serve four. Cut it into long slices, lengthwise, and spread the following mixture on both sides of each slice with a brush: 2 tablespoons of olive oil, a pinch each of salt and pepper, ½ teaspoon of Italian seasoning, 1 crushed clove of garlic, and 3 tablespoons of low-fat Italian dressing. If you want to take a shortcut, simply use regular Italian dressing that has olive oil as an ingredient. It won't be quite as good but is a bit easier. Grill the eggplant slices for about 5 minutes on each side over a medium-hot grill—just about the same amount of time you'd cook a piece of fish.

CAULIFLOWER AND GOLDEN RAISINS

Once again, cauliflower isn't one of my favorite vegetables, but that's when it's served raw as crudités or simply boiled, boring, and tasteless, in my humble opinion. This recipe bursts with flavor, and I prefer highly flavorful foods.

1 cup golden raisins	2 tablespoons olive oil
¼ cup gin (or rum, brandy, or other spirits)	1 tablespoon balsamic vinegar
1 head cauliflower, cut into florets and leaves removed	2 cloves of garlic, peeled and minced
	¼ cup candied walnuts or pecans

Start by soaking the raisins in the gin or other spirits, making sure they're all covered. The longer they soak, the better. Prepare the cauliflower florets. Mix the oil, vinegar, and garlic. Boil the cauliflower in a shallow pan, barely covered with water. (Here's another opportunity to add ¼ teaspoon of salt substitute to the water to include more potassium in your diet.) Cover the pan and cook the cauliflower for 3 to 4 minutes after the water comes to a boil, or until barely tender when tested with a fork. Drain the water, remove the cauliflower, and put it aside. Now add the oil, vinegar, and garlic to the pan and heat this before adding the cauliflower. Sauté it just long enough for the garlic to become transparent. Mix in the nuts and serve.

BROCCOLI AND CHEESE SAUCE

Here's another way to add wonderful flavor to a vegetable that's a fabulous source of potassium. I think even the first President Bush, who famously hated broccoli, would like this recipe.

2 large heads of broccoli, cut into florets	1 cup low-fat cheddar cheese, shredded
¼ cup each celery and onion, finely minced	½ cup low-fat sour cream
1 tablespoon canola oil	pinch each of salt and pepper

Place the broccoli florets in a shallow pan, barely covered with water. Bring them to a boil, cover the pan, bring the heat down to a low simmer, and cook the broccoli until it's bright green and tender without being mushy. Meanwhile, sauté the celery and onion in the oil until the onion is transparent. Mix in the cheese and sour cream. Blend this into the sautéed celery and onion and add the pinch of salt and pepper. Slowly and gently warm the mixture until the cheese melts.

Drain the broccoli and spread the sauce over it on a serving platter. Get ready to receive compliments to the chef.

SIMPLE SWEET POTATO

A medium-size sweet potato with its skin provides about 950 mg of potassium. Why not regularly include this tasty vegetable in your diet?

You have two options here. One, you can make mashed sweet potatoes in the same way you'd use white potatoes. Even simpler, just poke a few holes in the sweet potato, pop it into the microwave oven for about 10 minutes, and serve it with a dab of margarine and another of low-fat sour cream.

Seafood

FISH IN FOIL

I especially love two things about this recipe. First, you can prepare it ahead of time so it's great for entertaining. Second, there are no pots or pans to clean up. It's also easy and foolproof.

4 whole trout, baby salmon, or
  other small fish (1 per person)
1 lemon
1 onion, sliced into thin rings
1 tomato, cut into eighths and
  seeded

2 celery stalks, chopped
¼ cup parsley, finely minced
¼ teaspoon Old Bay's seafood
  seasoning
salt and pepper

Rinse and pat the fish dry and place each one on a 12-inch-long sheet of aluminum foil. Divide all the ingredients except the lemon and place them inside the fish cavities; put any extra onion rings on the outside of the fish. Cut the lemon and squeeze juice into the cavities of the four fish. Wrap and seal the fish in the foil. Indoors, bake the foil packets for 15 minutes in a 375 degree F oven. Outdoors, place the fish packets in the middle of the grill, using the indirect heat method, and roast them for 15 minutes.

SKEWERED SHRIMP AND SCALLOPS

Enjoy this recipe indoors in the oven or outdoors on the grill. You can substitute chunks of fish for the scallops.

MARINADE
½ cup chicken broth
½ cup canola oil
1 tablespoon each: lime, lemon,
  orange juice, and cider vinegar
3 tablespoons parsley, finely
  minced
3 garlic cloves, peeled and minced
1 pinch each salt and pepper

SKEWERING INGREDIENTS
8 ounces large shrimp
8 ounces scallops or fish chunks
2 bell peppers, one green and one
  yellow or orange
1 medium onion, cut into
  chunks
4 small tomatoes, cut in half

Place all of the ingredients in the mixed marinade in a sealed plastic bag and refrigerate it for 2 to 3 hours. Skewer the seafood and veggies alternately. Grill the kebobs until the shrimp and scallops lose their translucency. Do not overcook these delicate foods.

BOUILLABAISSE

I got this recipe from a chef friend of mine from the south of France and I simplified it to save time. Yes, it still takes a bit of time and effort, but it's a great treat for a special occasion. You don't get much more festive than this. Serve it with some crusty French bread and a cold white wine.

16 ounces vegetable broth (or fish stock if it's available)

4 ounces clam juice

4 ounces white wine

2 bay leaves

2 celery stalks, chopped

1 fennel root, chopped (you can replace this with ½ teaspoon each fennel and anise seed)

1 large onion, chopped

3 medium carrots, peeled and chopped

4 garlic cloves, peeled and minced

¼ teaspoon each rosemary and thyme

½ teaspoon orange zest (shaving of orange peel without pulp)

6 whole black peppercorns

1 teaspoon salt (optional)

1 teaspoon salt substitute (for extra potassium)

1 pound assorted seafood of your choice (There's quite a bit of controversy as to whether true bouillabaisse has any crustaceans, but again, it's your choice. Use chunks of fish, shrimp, clams, or mussels, and perhaps crab or crayfish.)

Place all the ingredients except the seafood in a large pot, bring it to a boil, and simmer it for 30 minutes. Add the seafood and simmer everything for another 15 minutes.

BLACKENED CAJUN SALMON

Chef Paul Prudhomme created this dish, which became a national favorite throughout the United States. His original dish called for redfish, found in the Gulf of Mexico, but you can use salmon or another fish of your choice. This dish is spectacular when served outdoors with your guests watching you cook as smoke billows up from the grill. (It's not a good idea to do this indoors unless you have a very powerful cooktop hood.) You'll need a cast-iron skillet large enough to accommodate all the fish, unless you make it in two or more batches.

Place the skillet directly on the coals or on the grill of a gas grill and heat it until it's literally white hot.

As the skillet heats, rinse and pat dry 6 ounces per person of salmon or another fish. Dredge the fish fillets in the blackening seasoning (described further on) that you prepared earlier. (I make a large amount that I can use for several meals.) Place a teaspoon or so of margarine on each fillet. Then carefully drop the fillets into the heated skillet. Expect that billowing smoke! The fish will cook quickly, owing to the high heat. After about 3 minutes, place another dab of margarine on the top of each fillet and flip it with a spatula to cook the other side for about 2 minutes.

This is a spicy dish. Many people would say that's an understatement. Serve it with cold beer to soothe your tongue!

BLACKENING SEASONING
1 tablespoon paprika
1 teaspoon garlic powder
1 teaspoon cayenne pepper
1 teaspoon onion powder
2 teaspoons salt (or 1 teaspoon
salt mixed with 1 teaspoon salt
substitute)
¾ teaspoon ground black pepper
½ teaspoon ground thyme
½ teaspoon oregano
½ teaspoon dried basil

Smoothies: Meals in a Jug

I started drinking smoothies as a convenient way to have breakfast while heading to the golf course on weekends. Then I often threw one together when I was in a hurry to get to a morning meeting. Now I keep a few jugs in my refrigerator and enjoy them throughout the week. The flavor combinations are virtually limitless so I never tire of them and neither will you. This is an incredibly healthy habit to get into, since each smoothie contains three or four servings of fruit, many of which are excellent sources of magnesium and potassium, and nonfat milk provides both calcium and potassium. It's one of the best ways to balance your electrolytes, negating the effects of sodium in your diet.

One medium banana, a staple ingredient in all my smoothie recipes, has 467 mg of potassium; cantaloupe provides 547 mg per cup; a medium mango gives you 323 mg; a medium pear has 208 mg; 8 ounces of orange juice (or frozen concentrate to reconstitute to that amount) has 436 mg; 8 ounces of grape juice offers 334 mg. An 8-ounce serving of nonfat milk has 407 mg of potassium along with 301 mg of calcium. A smoothie made from milk, orange juice, a banana, a mango, and a pear would add up to a whopping 1,627 mg of potassium! (By the way, if you're looking for the potassium champion of the fruit world, that would be the durian [they say it tastes like heaven and stinks like hell] with 1,059 mg per cup.) That's not counting all the fiber and other nutrients. A smoothie of that size, typical of what I bring to the golf course, will satisfy you for most of the day until your afternoon snack or an early dinner.

I've included quite a few of my favorite recipes, frequently spiked with cocoa powder or grape juice concentrate to provide lots of flavor as well as a load of blood pressure–healthy polyphenols. Look to berries for even more polyphenols. There's no limit to the combinations of ingredients. On a happy, economical note, you'll never waste fruit when it gets a bit overripe!

When certain fruits, such as mangos and peaches, are in season, I buy them at their best taste and lowest price, let them get nice and ripe, and store them in packets in the freezer. Many stores also stock bags of frozen fruits and berries. I keep frozen orange juice and red grape juice concentrate handy as well. Egg substitute is an excellent protein source to balance the meal's nutritional profile. If your smoothie comes out thicker than you'd like, just add more milk, water, or juice to thin it out to your preference.

I add a scoop of Profibe, a concentrated source of the soluble fiber pectin, to every one of my smoothies. Profibe is completely odorless and tasteless, and you'll never notice it in the smoothies you consume, but the soluble fiber will help you to keep your cholesterol under control.

BASIC SMOOTHIE

This smoothie has 540 calories, a very reasonable amount for break-fast or lunch.

8 ounces water (or use orange juice if you have it in the refrigerator)

8 ounces nonfat milk (80 calories)

2 ounces frozen orange juice concentrate (130 calories)

4 ounces egg substitute (60 calories) (never consume raw eggs, owing to salmonella risk)

1 cup frozen mixed berries (70 calories)

1 medium banana (100 calories)

1 medium pear (100 calories)

1 scoop Profibe

Preparation is simply a matter of putting all the ingredients into a blender and whirling them into a delicious mixture. I make two to three smoothies at a time for convenience and keep them in jugs in the refrigerator for when I need a quick, on-the-run meal.

CREAMSICLE SMOOTHIE

I've named this for a frozen confection of vanilla ice cream and orange sherbet on a stick that was very popular when I was a child and is still sold today. It's delicious and refreshing.

8 ounces water

8 ounces nonfat milk

2 ounces frozen orange juice con-centrate

4 ounces egg substitute

1 medium banana

1 medium orange, peeled and seeded

1 tablespoon honey

½ teaspoon vanilla extract

1 scoop Profibe

FUDGSICLE SMOOTHIE

Yup, this one's named after another frozen confection on a stick. It takes advantage of the high polyphenol content of plain cocoa pow-der (not hot cocoa mix).

8 ounces water
8 ounces nonfat milk
4 ounces egg substitute
1 medium banana
1 medium mango (replace with
    raspberries for variety and a
    special taste treat)

1 tablespoon honey (more if
    you prefer it sweeter; you
    can also use artificial
    sweetener)
2 tablespoons cocoa powder
1 scoop Profibe

STRAWBERRY SCREAMER

I live in a part of California that's famous for strawberries. There's a strawberry festival every spring. When strawberries are in season, I buy them by the flat, gorge like a bear, and freeze bags of them for another time.

8 ounces water
8 ounces nonfat milk
4 ounces egg substitute
2 ounces frozen white grape juice
1 medium banana

2 cups fresh or frozen
    strawberries
2 tablespoons cocoa powder
1 scoop Profibe

BANANA BLUEBERRY BONANZA

Of all the berries, blueberries have the highest antioxidant potential. Once again, whenever they're in season, I have my fill and freeze the rest for the future.

8 ounces water
8 ounces nonfat milk
2 ounces frozen red grape juice
    concentrate (this goes well
    with all berry smoothies)

4 ounces egg substitute
2 medium bananas
1 cup fresh or frozen blueberries
    (or more if you prefer, as I do)
1 scoop Profibe

PURPLE COW

When I was a kid, my Mom used to mix a glass of milk with grape juice, calling it a purple cow. This smoothie has all that flavor and more nutritional value.

8 ounces water
8 ounces nonfat milk
4 ounces egg substitute
2 or 3 ounces frozen red grape
   juice concentrate

1 cup seedless red or black
   grapes
1 medium banana
1 scoop Profibe

CHOCOLATE PEANUT BUTTER CUP

That candy confection is one of my favorites, but I avoid it because of the saturated fat. So I came up with this smoothie to satisfy my craving. The peanut butter adds some healthy fat and the extra calories keep away the hungries for a long time.

8 ounces water
8 ounces nonfat milk
1 medium banana
1 medium pear
4 ounces egg substitute
2 ounces frozen orange juice
   concentrate

2 or 3 tablespoons peanut
   butter
2 tablespoons honey
2 heaping tablespoons cocoa
   powder
1 scoop Profibe

MELON MADNESS

This isn't really a smoothie as much as it is a fruit slurry. Call it what you want, it's a cold, refreshing, and nourishing drink during the summer melon season.

8 ounces orange juice
2 cups cantaloupe chunks
2 cups honeydew melon chunks

2 cups seedless watermelon
   chunks
2 tablespoons honey

Desserts and Treats

Here are more opportunities to incorporate fruit into your diet in delicious ways far beyond simply gnawing on an apple or peeling a banana. Preparation is remarkably simple and takes little time.

BANANAS FLAMBÉ WITHOUT THE FLAME

The original recipe, which you can duplicate if you feel like getting fancy some evening, calls for adding a tablespoon of banana liqueur and a tablespoon of brandy to the melted margarine and sugar, heating this, and then igniting it with a match to yield a spectacular effect. If you'd like the taste of the liqueur and brandy without the flame, you can simply add them to the skillet and heat them for a while without igniting them.

1 tablespoon tub margarine
1 tablespoon brown sugar

2 bananas sliced lengthwise
low-fat vanilla ice cream

Melt the margarine in a skillet and add the brown sugar at low heat. Stir this until the sugar melts and blends with the margarine. Sauté and brown the bananas. Serve them with a scoop of ice cream for each banana. Serves two people.

CARAMEL APPLES ON A PLATE
INSTEAD OF A STICK

1 apple per person
1 tablespoon low-fat or nonfat
  caramel ice cream topping

2 tablespoons walnuts, chopped

Slice the apple and place the slices on a plate. Drizzle them with the caramel topping. Top them with chopped walnuts.

BROILED OR GRILLED PINEAPPLE

Pineapple can often be quite tart, unless you happen to be enjoying it on a tropical island where the fruit grows and it's picked at its perfect ripeness. Heating the pineapple—in this case, grilling it—breaks down the starch into natural sugars and releases a wonderful sweet flavor.

1 pineapple, sliced as wheels

maple syrup, honey, or brown
  sugar

Arrange the pineapple wheels on a broiling pan and drizzle them with your preferred sweetener. Broil them until they're browned. You can also grill them over the coals outdoors.

RASPBERRIES AND CHAMBORD LIQUEUR

This is an elegant dessert idea for entertaining. Serve each person a plate on which you place a small bowl of fresh, rinsed raspberries (they're best when they're in season), a shot glass of Chambord raspberry liqueur, and a toothpick. Use the toothpick to pierce and pick up a raspberry to dip as a "cup" into the liqueur. You'll get raves for this no-effort presentation.

MANGO WITH STICKY RICE

1 large mango, peeled and sliced, for two people
2 cups cooked Japanese sticky rice (it's even better when made with low-fat coconut milk or half coconut milk and half water), warm not hot

This short list tells it all. Just arrange the mango slices on one side of a small dessert plate and the warm rice on the other. The combined tastes are marvelous. You may see this dessert on an upscale Thai restaurant menu.

FRUIT AND CHEESE PLATTER

This is the ultimate European dessert, enjoyed far more frequently by the French and other Europeans than elaborate dishes are. You need just a little of the intensely flavored cheeses suggested here to offset the sweetness of the fruit. One-half ounce of cheese has just over 4 grams of fat. The following recipe serves two.

1 apple
1 pear
1 cup grapes
1 ounce blue, cheddar, or brie cheese

Thinly slice the apple and pear and for each person, arrange half of each type of fruit slices in fans on a platter with a half cup of grapes and a half ounce of cheese. Try this with a glass of full-bodied red wine.

PEACH MELBA

Here's a flashback to the fifties. If you're younger than fifty-five you may never have heard of it. Either way, just reading the following recipe is sure to get your taste buds revved up.

This is a variation on the classic recipe, eliminating the brandy added to the skillet to flame the dessert. You can do that if you wish, but it's really not necessary.

¼ cup raspberry preserves	1 teaspoon lemon juice
3 tablespoons brown sugar	low-fat vanilla ice cream
½ cup water	2 cups fresh raspberries
4 large peaches, peeled, pitted, and sliced	

Combine the preserves, sugar, and water in a skillet and simmer them over low heat until they're syrupy, about 5 minutes. Add the peaches and cook them for another 3 to 4 minutes, turning them a few times until they're tender. (Out of season, you can use frozen peaches.) Add the lemon juice and stir it through.

Divide the cooked peaches onto four saucers and top each one with a small scoop of ice cream. Spoon the syrupy sauce over the peaches and ice cream. Top each dish with raspberries.

DAWN'S GOOEY CHOCOLATE CAKE

My wife, Dawn, is a far better baker than I am, since she likes to follow recipes to the letter and I tend to wing it. Baking calls for strict adherence to directions, but this recipe is easy enough even for me to follow without messing it up. Even so, it tastes better when Dawn makes this cake for me—it's the love factor. Beyond the sheer indulgence, you'll get the polyphenols of cocoa and the good fats, omega-3 fatty acids, of walnuts. Dawn modified this recipe from the original 1969 Betty Crocker's Cookbook *that both of us use more than any other cookbook in our rather large library.*

1 cup flour (if you're feeling really healthy, you can use whole-grain flour)
¾ cup granulated sugar
2 tablespoons cocoa powder (not hot cocoa mix)
2 teaspoons baking powder
¼ teaspoon salt

½ cup nonfat milk
2 tablespoons tub margarine, melted but not hot in microwave oven
1 cup walnuts, chopped
1 cup brown sugar, packed
¼ cup cocoa powder
1¾ cups hot water

Preheat the oven to 350 degrees F. Blend the flour, granulated sugar, 2 tablespoons of cocoa powder, baking powder, and salt in a mixing bowl. Add the milk and margarine and stir in the walnuts. Pour the mixture into an ungreased 9 × 9 × 2-inch-square pan. Mix the brown sugar and ¼ cup of cocoa powder and sprinkle this over the batter in the pan. Pour the hot water over the batter. Bake it for 45 minutes.

You'll wind up with a wonderful combination of cake and pudding. Cut the cake topped with pudding into squares for serving. We like to garnish it with low-fat whipped cream or vanilla ice cream. Make this once and it'll become one of your favorites.

CHOCOLATE BANANA PUDDING

Here's a dessert that combines the blood pressure benefits of potassium in a banana with the polyphenols of cocoa.

Slice a ripe banana into either instant or regular (cooked) nonfat chocolate pudding mix. Conversely, mix 2 heaping tablespoons of cocoa powder into nonfat pudding mix; you can also slice in a banana.

BLOOD PRESSURE–LOWERING HOT COCOA

Ever since I learned the benefits of cocoa's polyphenols, I've gotten into the habit of frequently sipping a cup of hot cocoa in the evening.

It's a soothing, relaxing, and healthful ritual before bedtime. The following recipe is for one mug, one serving, but you can multiply it for more than one person.

Heat 1 cup of nonfat milk in the microwave oven. Put 2 tablespoons of dark cocoa and one tablespoon of sugar or the equivalent of artificial sweetener into a mug. Pour the heated milk into the mug and stir. Top the mug with a few mini-marshmallows for a treat.

Here are a few alternative hot cocoa flavors. Just add one of the following to the blend:

Add 1 tablespoon of raspberry jam or orange marmalade, 1 tablespoon of frozen red grape or orange juice concentrate, 1 teaspoon of vanilla extract, or 1 teaspoon of instant coffee (decaf at bedtime). Or add a pinch of cinnamon or nutmeg, or both. Also experiment with flavor concentrates, such as orange, lemon, or rum extract.

NEW YORK EGG CREAM

To the uninitiated, this beverage must contain egg and cream, right? Wrong. How it got its name is a matter of conjecture, but it's a delicious treat from Brooklyn and is served in delis throughout the United States and even outside the country.

The original recipe calls for 2 tablespoons of chocolate syrup, ½ cup of whole milk, and 1 cup of seltzer water, but I've modified that significantly in an equally delicious alternative that packs more of cocoa's polyphenols and eliminates the sodium from seltzer water.

In a large glass, mix 2 tablespoons of chocolate syrup and 1 tablespoon of cocoa powder until the cocoa is completely blended. Next add 4 ounces of cold nonfat milk and stir. Now add 4 ounces of cold club soda (sparkling water) followed by another 4 ounces of cold milk. Stir it gently to save the bubbles. Serve it with ice cubes or plain, and sip it through a straw for authenticity.

18

Take the Pressure Off
Your Heart

I nearly forgot to mention the most important weapons to lower blood pressure and prevent cardiovascular disease, heart attack, and stroke. You've read about ways to cope with stress, lose weight, quit smoking cigarettes, become more physically active, improve your diet, and counterbalance salt and sodium. You've learned about natural, safe, and clinically documented effective supplements that can dramatically lower both systolic and diastolic blood pressure. Those supplements weren't even available when I was first inspired to write this book after studying newly published blood pressure guidelines in 2003. So what's missing?

If some company could bottle the ingredients that virtually guarantee success in blood pressure control and heart disease prevention, doctors worldwide would write prescriptions and the company would make countless millions of dollars and euros and pounds and yen. But no one ever will because those truly secret ingredients can be found only in your own heart and soul. They are motivation and commitment.

It has now been well over two decades since that cardiac surgeon told me that the second bypass operation I needed might kill me, leaving my children without their daddy. If some mysterious supernatural being came into my apartment that day when I wept at the thought of my wife having to tell little Ross and Jenny that

Daddy's never coming home from the hospital, I would have jumped at any deal offered. I would have gladly accepted death the day they were off to college if it meant I could see them grow to that degree of independence. My kids were my motivation and the source of my continued commitment through the years.

Of course, it turned out that I didn't have to sign that sort of contract, and it's a good thing, too. I've lived to see Ross and Jenny grow up into fine young adults who are well on their way to productive careers. I've outlived my father by many years. My cardiologist calls my test results superb. And the year this book is published I become eligible for Medicare! Wow, I never expected to live this long.

But now I've gotten greedy! Life has never been better or sweeter. I love my wife, Dawn, and we're looking forward to growing older together and enjoying some of the rewards of decades of hard work, such as travel, and savoring the simple joys of reading books, watching sunsets, and marveling at the beauty of a flower or a bird or a mountain. Ross and Jenny still like to ask my advice on personal and professional matters. And I want to be around for the day when my first grandchild is born and I get to hold him or her in my arms, to witness again all those wonderful stages of childhood, and dole out the love I have in my heart. Lord, how I wish my dad had that chance. Sadly he did not, but I do. The realization for those hopes and dreams in the future, sharing life with my wonderful family, remain my motivation and commitment.

But enough about me! What about you? What are the reasons for your motivation and commitment to health? What are your reasons for taking the pressure off your heart by lowering your blood pressure? What will inspire you to take that brisk walk when you'd rather watch TV? To make food choices based on other than taste alone? To lose those extra pounds and put out that last cigarette? To religiously take those supplements? Only you have the incredible power to choose a long and healthy life—or should I say to *work* for that life.

Most men and women never really stop, as the old proverb goes, to smell the roses. They don't even bother to look at them. Close your eyes for a moment. Think about all the true joys in your life. Your family. Your career. Your hobbies. Your religious beliefs. Do you love to fish? To hike? To cook? What will be *your* motivation?

Even more than when I first began to write this book, I now know that the program in these pages really works. Readers of my quarterly publication, *The Diet-Heart Newsletter*, had an advance opportunity to try the program for themselves before the book came even close to publication. Every time I got a report of success from them, I felt not selfish pride but gratitude that I could share this information. Doctors who have incorporated the program in their practices tell me over and over about how their patients have benefited.

But no program will do any good until you make it a part of your own life. No drug company or supplement maker will put motivation and commitment into pills or tablets or capsules for you to swallow.

A frequent theme in literature and in movies involves a person seeing the world after his or her death. Think Dickens's *A Christmas Carol*, and Jimmy Stewart in *It's a Wonderful Life*. Now think about the world without you. Imagine the tears of your loved ones. Picture yourself not being able to do all the things you've wanted to do. Four decades later, I still miss my father. My wife and children would certainly miss me. And many would miss you.

The time to ensure a long, healthy, happy life is now. Find that motivation deep inside your inner self to take the pressure off your heart starting today. For tomorrow, and tomorrow, and tomorrow. Join me in the celebration of heart health!

References

1. Hypertension: The Silent Killer

American Journal of Kidney Diseases, March 2003.
American Journal of Medicine, February 2006.
Annals of Family Medicine, July-August 2005.
Annals of Internal Medicine, April 5, 2006.
British Medical Journal, June 2001.
Circulation, June 18, 2002.
Hypertension Management Guide for Doctors, 2004, Heart Foundation of Australia.
Journal of the American Medical Association, May 14, 2003.
Journal of the American Medical Association (JNC7 Report), May 21, 2003.
The Lancet, November 17, 2001.
New England Journal of Medicine, November 1, 2001.
New England Journal of Medicine, March 15, 2006.
New England Journal of Medicine, April 20, 2006.
Proceedings of the American College of Cardiology, March 2006.
Stroke, February 2006.

2. Testing Your Pressure

American Journal of Hypertension, February 4, 2004.
Archives of Internal Medicine, July 11, 2005.
Circulation, March 18, 2003.
Hypertension, December 30, 2005.
Journal of the American Medical Association, May 31, 2003.

3. Different Blood Pressure Concerns for Different People

American College of Cardiology Annual Scientific Sessions, 2004.
American Heart Association: Heart Facts, 2003.
Circulation, November 21, 2005.
Circulation, January 30, 2006.
Journal of the American Medical Association, May 5, 2004.
Journal of the American Medical Association, July 27, 2005.
Journal Watch Cardiology, November 23, 2005.
Medscape Cardiology, Hypertension Highlights, November 11, 2003.
Medscape Cardiology, April 5, 2005.
National High Blood Pressure Education Program Working Group on High
    Blood Pressure in Children and Adolescents, 2004.

Pediatrics June 2004.
Proceedings of the American Society of Nephrology Annual Meeting, November
    2005.
Stroke, May 2006.

4. Blood Pressure and Diabetes

British Journal of Diabetes and Vascular Disease, March 2006.
Circulation, February 3, 2004.
Circulation, March 27, 2006.
Diabetes Care, March 2004.
"Diabetes & Cardiovascular Disease Review: Hypertension in Diabetes," a publi-
    cation of the American Diabetes Association/American College of Cardiology,
    2002.
Hypertension, March 2006.
Journal of the American Medical Association, October 8, 2003.
Life Sciences, October 2004.
Medscape Cardiology, October 19, 2005.

5. Weight and Blood Pressure

American Journal of Clinical Nutrition, March 2004.
American Journal of Clinical Nutrition, June 2005.
American Journal of Hypertension, May 2004.
Annals of Internal Medicine, January 3, 2006.
Archives of Internal Medicine, June 13, 2005.
Circulation, January 31, 2006.
Environmental Nutrition, February 2006.
Food Values of Portions Commonly Used, 17th ed., Jean A. T. Pennington, New
    York: Lippincott Williams & Wilkins, 2005.
Journal of the American Medical Association, January 4, 2006.
The Lancet, November 5, 2005.
Medical Journal of Australia, November-December 2003.

6. Enjoy a Pressure-Friendly Active Lifestyle

Annals of Internal Medicine, April 2002.
Circulation, September 18, 2001.
Circulation, February 18, 2003.
Circulation, July 26, 2005.
The Lancet, October 8, 2005.
Preventive Medicine, September 2005.

7. Reduce Your Stress

American Journal of Hypertension, July 16, 2001.
British Medical Journal (online first), January 19, 2006.
Circulation, May 20, 2002.
Circulation, March 23, 2004.
Journal of Clinical Hypertension, August 4, 2004.
Medical Journal of Australia (Stress Position Statement), 2003.

Proceedings of the Scientific Sessions of the American Heart Association, November 2005.
Stroke, August 3, 2001.

9. Balance Your Electrolytes: Sodium, Potassium, Calcium, and Magnesium

Sodium

British Medical Journal, September 21, 2002.
Hypertension, June 7, 1995.
Journal of Clinical Hypertension, July 14, 2004.
The Lancet, January 14, 2006.

Potassium

American Journal of Clinical Nutrition, June 2006.
Annals of Internal Medicine, July 15, 1991.
British Journal of Nutrition, July 2003.
Food Values of Portions Commonly Used, 17th ed., Jean A. T. Pennington, New York: Lippincott Williams & Wilkins, 2005.
Hypertension, January 24, 2005.
Hypertension, April 12, 2005.
Proceedings of the American Heart Association, November 1994.

Calcium

American Journal of Hypertension, October 24, 2003.
Proceedings of the American Heart Association, November 1992.

Magnesium

American Journal of Cardiology, October 10, 2003.
American Journal of Hypertension, August 21, 2002.
Circulation, April 4, 2006.
Medscape Medical News, January 8, 2004.

10. Drink, but Not Too Much

American Journal of Geriatric Cardiology, June 2005.
American Journal of Hypertension, October 19, 2005.
American Journal of Hypertension, February 2006.
Archives of Internal Medicine, March 22, 2004.
British Medical Journal, January 20, 2006.
Circulation, September 6, 2005.
Hypertension, January 23, 2006.
The Lancet, December 3, 2005.
Stroke, January 18, 2006.
Stroke, January 25, 2006.

11. Lower Your Cholesterol, Lower Your Blood Pressure

American Journal of Clinical Nutrition, November 2005.
American Journal of Clinical Nutrition, April 2006.

Archives of Internal Medicine, November 14, 2005.

Circulation, June 1997.

Circulation, November 1999.

European Heart Journal, September 2005.

Hypertension, January 2006.

Journal of the American Medical Association, November 16, 2005.

New England Journal of Medicine, September 22, 2005.

Proceedings of the American Heart Association Annual Scientific Sessions, November 2005.

Stroke, January 1997.

12. Eating to Lower Blood Pressure

Chocolate

Hypertension, July 18, 2005.

Coffee and Tea

Archives of Internal Medicine, July 26, 2004.

Journal of the American College of Cardiology, January 17, 2006.

Journal of the American Medical Association, November 9, 2005.

Effects of Diet on Blood Pressure

American Journal of Clinical Nutrition, February 2006.

Archives of Internal Medicine, January 9, 2006.

Diabetes Care, December 2005.

Hypertension, May 19, 2003.

Journal of Clinical Hypertension, April 2005.

The Lancet, January 28, 2006.

Omega-3 Fatty Acids

American Heart Association Scientific Statement, November 19, 2002.

American Journal of Clinical Nutrition, January 2003.

Circulation, August 19, 2003.

Circulation, September 27, 2005.

New England Journal of Medicine, November 28, 2002.

13. Daily Blood Pressure Busters

Acupuncture

Abstracts of the American Heart Association Scientific Sessions, 2005.

Arginine

Alternative Medicine Review, March 2002.

American Journal of Nutrition, March 2000.

International Journal of Cardiology, February 2002.

Journal of the American College of Nutrition, February 2002.

Journal of Nutrition, December 2000.

Aspirin

Journal of the American Medical Association, January 18, 2006.

New England Journal of Medicine, March 7, 2005.
Proceedings of the Annual Conference on Arteriosclerosis, Thrombosis, and Vascular Biology, 2004.

Breathing

High-blood-pressure-help.com.
Medscape Cardiology, July 25, 2002.

Co-Enzyme Q10

Journal of Human Hypertension, February 1999.
Naturaldatabase.com, February 2003.
Pharmacotherapy, May 2001.
Southern Medical Journal, July 2001.

Eye Examinations

British Journal of Ophthalmology, March 2005.
British Journal of Ophthalmology, August 2005.
Hypertension, August 2004.

Fermented Milk

American Journal of Hypertension, January 2006.

Fish Oil

Alternative Medical Review, April 2001.
Medscape Cardiology, June 2004.
Naturaldatabase.com, February 2003.
Prostaglandins, Leucotrienes and Essential Fatty Acids, January 1999.

Folic Acid

American Journal of Clinical Nutrition, July 2005.
Proceedings of the American Heart Association Council for High Blood Pressure Research, 2004.
Stroke, September 2005.

Garlic

Archives of Internal Medicine, April 2001.
Journal of Hypertension, March 1994.
Journal of Nutrition, (Supplement), 2001.
Naturaldatabase.com, February 2003.

Herbs

MayoClinic.com, November 2005.
Phytotherapy Research, January 2002.

Laughter

Heart, February 2006.

Loneliness

Psychology and Aging, March 2006.

Melatonin

American Journal of Hypertension, December 2005.
Hypertension, January 2004.

Music

British Medical Journal, September 2001.
Heart, October 2005.

Over-the-Counter and Prescription Drugs

American Journal of Medicine, September 2005.
Archives of Internal Medicine, August 2005.
Consumerlab.com, November 2005.
Heart Foundation (Australia): Non-Drug Management of Hypertension, September 2004.
MayoClinic.com, November 2005.

Sleep Disorders

Current Cardiology Reports, November 2005.
Current Hypertension Reports, October 2003.
Hypertension, February 3, 2006.
Hypertension, April 3, 2006.
Hypertension, May 4, 2006.

Vitamins

Alternative Medicine Review, April 2001.
The Lancet, December 1999.
Naturaldatabase.com, February 2003.

14. The Blood Pressure Cure 5 Secret Weapons

Arginine

Alternative Medicine Review, January 2005.
American Journal of Cardiology, October 10, 2005.
British Journal of Pharmacology, January 2006.
Canadian Journal of Physiology and Pharmacology, August-September 2005.
Circulation (Abstracts of the American Heart Association Scientific Sessions), November 2006.
Journal of the American Medical Association, January 4, 2006.
Personal correspondence: Lance Gould, M.D., University of Texas.
Recent Progress in Medicine (Italian), October 2005.
Vascular Medicine, July 2005.
Vascular Medicine, November 2005.

Chocolate and Cocoa

American Journal of Clinical Nutrition, January 2005.
Archives of Internal Medicine, February 27, 2006.
Hypertension, August 2005.
Pharmaceutical Business Review, March 2006.
Proceedings of the National Academy of Sciences, January 24, 2006.

Grape Seed Extract

Abstracts of the 219th American Chemical Society National Meeting, March 2000.
Abstracts of the 225th American Chemical Society National Meeting, March 2006.
Abstracts of the Experimental Biology Conference, April 2005.
American Journal of Clinical Nutrition, May 2002.
American Journal of Clinical Nutrition (Supplement), January 2005.
Bottom Line Health, January 2004.
Chemical Innovation, September 2000.
Circulation, June 18, 2002.
Environmental Nutrition, May 2004.
European Journal of Clinical Pharmacology, February 2006.
Journal of Medicinal Food, November 1, 2001.

Lycopene and Tomato Extract

Abstracts of the American Chemical Society Annual Meeting, March 2006.
American Heart Journal, January 2006.
American Journal of Clinical Nutrition (Supplement), January 2005.
Biochemistry and Biophysics Research Communications, April 28, 1997.

Pycnogenol

European Bulletin of Drug Research, July 1999.
Evidence-Based Integrative Medicine, August 2003.
Journal of Cardiovascular Pharmacology, March 1998.
Life Sciences, June 2004.
Nutrition Research, September 2001.

16. Understanding Prescription Drugs: The Last Resort to Lowering Blood Pressure

American College of Cardiology Internet search.
American Heart Association Internet search.
Circulation, May 2, 2006.
Journal of the American Medical Association, September 2002.
Journal of the American Medical Association, May 21, 2003.
Journal of Hypertension, June 2003.
The Lancet, November 6, 2004.
The Lancet, September 10, 2005.
Medscape Cardiology Internet search.
New England Journal of Medicine, January 20, 2000.
Pharmacotherapy, November 2005.

Index